In
Blinding Pain

A Rainbow Book

"*Blinding Pain, Simple Truth* is an intriguing blend of Buddhist insight meditation and a fascinating interpretation of key Hebrew Bible passages. In this engaging work, Dr. Richard Ellis shares his own journey of life-changing transformation through these liberating practices and studies. The pairing of these two ancient traditions helps to illuminate our own explorations of healing and awakening."

—Joseph Goldstein, author of *A Heart Full of Peace* and *One Dharma: The Emerging Western Buddhism*

"Physical pain is sometimes unavoidable, but suffering is a choice. Sounds nice, but is it true? And if it is true, what choices does a person have to make to find freedom and perhaps even fulfillment in the midst of severe and persistent pain? The book you have in your hand is a rich, informative, and empowering narrative of one person's quest for happiness, independent of conditions. It is informative and empowering because it details step-by-step the sequence of challenges and breakthroughs that the author went through over a period of many years. It is rich because it brings together three deep human endeavors: Buddhist mindfulness practice, higher mathematics, and traditional Jewish text study.

"Delicious for the intellect, nourishing for the soul."

—Shinzen Young, author of *The Science of Enlightenment* and *Break Through Pain*

"Professor Richard Ellis invites us, as fellow human beings, to join him on his intimate personal journey to discover the heart of reality: when we experience pain and our lives are afflicted by suffering, we can experience healing and transformation. Personal pain, which can challenge our notions of self and our conventional view of the world, can also become our teacher....

"Richard enriches his journey of self-discovery and transformation by celebrating Hebrew Scripture and ancient Buddhist wisdom. Archetypal Biblical ancestors come alive as Richard explores their struggles, which are our own.... Buddhist wisdom complements the wisdom of Hebrew Scripture by offering us the gift of meditation, which allows us to experience the fullness of reality itself.

"I am profoundly grateful to Richard for sharing his book with me at a time of personal transition. As a former hospital chaplain, I engaged human suffering on many levels. I humbly bow to Richard's embrace of pain, reality, and God's mystery. All who read this book will be enriched by Richard's witness."

—Father Bruce Teague, Our Lady of the Valley Church, Sheffield, MA

"Richard Ellis's close account of his struggle with physical pain opens up very useful insights into the nature of suffering and the role of the ego in prolonging it. For him, pain has become a kind of teacher, and the story of his journey to understand the teaching of his pain brings into one book his knowledge as a mathematician, as a close reader of the Hebrew Bible, and as a practitioner of Buddhist meditation."

—RODGER KAMENETZ, AUTHOR OF *THE JEW IN THE LOTUS: A POET'S REDISCOVERY OF JEWISH IDENTITY IN BUDDHIST INDIA*

"I encourage both laypersons and professionals to read this unique integration of Buddhism, the Bible, and behavioral science. The author uses Buddhist teachings, meditation, the wisdom of the Bible, and his own experiences to explore issues of pain and suffering, healing and happiness, ego and enlightenment. The book describes a path of transformation: how people focused on achievement and control can discover a new way of being, based on insight and love. Such a transformation is exactly what we are striving for in biofeedback, cognitive behavior therapy, and modern psychoanalysis."

—DR. ARNON ROLNICK, CLINICAL PSYCHOLOGIST AND SENIOR RESEARCH FELLOW, UNIT FOR APPLIED NEUROSCIENCE, INTERDISCIPLINARY CENTER, AND PSYCHOTHERAPY SCHOOL, BEN GURION UNIVERSITY, ISRAEL

"This is a rich and rewarding book that shares deep insights about life, human suffering and ways to cope with it, meditation, and texts from the Jewish Bible. They are delivered compellingly, poetically, and often with an element of humor. The author's wisdom and clarity of thought comes shining through, whether his mode is story-telling memoirist, scholarly analyst, spiritual guide, or self-help coach. I recommend this book highly to anyone seeking help with intractable physical, emotional, or spiritual pain."

—KENNETH TALAN, M.D., AUTHOR OF THE AWARD-WINNING BOOK, *HELP YOUR CHILD OR TEEN GET BACK ON TRACK: WHAT PARENTS AND PROFESSIONALS CAN DO FOR CHILDHOOD EMOTIONAL AND BEHAVIORAL PROBLEMS*

"This book is a mindful and wholehearted exploration of the nature of pain, suffering, and healing that reveals surprising discoveries of simple, yet challenging pathways to equanimity. It also presents imaginative and evocative interpretations of Biblical narratives and their relationship to Buddha Dharma, meditative practice, and wisdom."

—TED SLOVIN, PH.D., FORMER MEMBER OF THE BOARD OF DIRECTORS OF THE INSIGHT MEDITATION SOCIETY, BARRE, MA; PSYCHOLOGIST

Blinding Pain, Simple Truth
Changing Your Life Through Buddhist Meditation

Richard S. Ellis

Rainbow Books, Inc.
FLORIDA

Library of Congress Cataloging-In-Publication Data

Ellis, Richard S. (Richard Steven), 1947–
 Blinding pain, simple truth : changing your life through Buddhist meditation / Richard S. Ellis. — 1st ed.
   p. cm.
 Includes bibliographical references.
 ISBN 978-1-56825-125-7 (trade softcover : alk. paper)
 1. Meditation—Buddhism. 2. Suffering—Religious aspects—Buddhism. 3. Pain—Religious aspects—Buddhism. 4. Suffering in the Bible. 5. Ellis, Richard S. (Richard Steven), 1947– 6. Spiritual biography—United States. 7. Headache patients' writings. I. Title.
 BQ5612.E45 2011
 294.3'4435—dc22
                          2010003580

Blinding Pain, Simple Truth:
Changing Your Life Through Buddhist Meditation
Copyright © 2011 Richard S. Ellis

ISBN-10: 1-56825-125-4 • ISBN-13: 978-1-56825-125-7

Published by
Rainbow Books, Inc., PO Box 430, Highland City, FL 33846-0430

Editorial Offices and Wholesale/Distributor Orders
Telephone: (863) 648-4420 • Email: RBIbooks@aol.com • *www.RainbowBooksInc.com*

Individuals' Orders
BCH Distribution (800) 431-1579 • *www.BookCH.com*
www.AllBookStores.com • *www.Amazon.com*

Retailers' Orders
BCH Distribution • Ingram Book Company • Baker & Taylor Books

All rights reserved. No part of this book may be reproduced or transmitted in any form or by any means, electronic or mechanical (except as follows for photocopying for review purposes). Permission for photocopying can be obtained for internal or personal use, the internal or personal use of specific clients, and for educational use, by paying the appropriate fee to

Copyright Clearance Center, 222 Rosewood Dr.
Danvers, MA 01923 U.S.A.

Disclaimer: The information contained in this publication is not intended to serve as a replacement for professional assistance. Any use of the information in this publication is at the reader's discretion. The author and the publisher specifically disclaim any and all liability arising directly or indirectly from the use or application of any information contained herein. A competent professional should be consulted regarding your specific situation. Further, the author and/or publisher have not and will not receive any financial consideration for any recommendation of various sources provided that have items such as services and/or goods of any kind for sale. Further still, references are made to a number of Internet sites; at the time of writing, these sites did not contain, to the best of the author's and/or the publisher's knowledge, material that might be offensive to general standards of decency.

The paper used in this publication meets the minimum requirements of the American National Standard for Information Sciences—Permanence of Paper for Printed Library Materials, ANSI Z39.48-1984.

First Edition 2011
15 14 13 12 11   7 6 5 4 3 2 1
Printed in the United States of America.

For Alison,

for Melissa, Ken, Noah, and Lilah,

and for Michael and Lauren.

May God protect you. May you be safe.

May God enlighten you. May you be enlightened.

May you see God's face in every face you see and thus find peace.

Contents

Preface   ix

Introduction   1

Headaches and Healing
    1. Letting Go of the Past   19
    2. Our Wounds Will Heal Us   37
    3. Waking Up to the Truth   55

Buddhist Lessons from the Bible
    4. Face to Face with Jacob   93
    5. Conceptual Thinking Banishes Us from Eden   125
    6. Becoming Job: Going Beyond Words   157

Today
    7. What Pain Can Teach Us   171
    8. Finding Equanimity on the Massachusetts Turnpike   207

Appendix: Learning to Meditate   213

Bibliography   217

Suggested Reading   227

About the Author   233

We set up a word at the point at which our ignorance begins, at which we can see no further, e.g., the word "I," the word "do," the word "suffer": — these are perhaps the horizon of our knowledge, but not "truths."

— JOHN BANVILLE, *Shroud*

Restraint is for this: to see the difference between pain and suffering. Pain is inevitable, but suffering is not. Suffering arises when I fight the world's lawfulness, the dharma. When I desire things to arise differently from how they do arise, there is suffering. When I desire that things which arise not pass away, there is suffering.

— SHARON CAMERON, *Beautiful Work: A Meditation on Pain*

The challenge must be to come unstuck, resist habit — the same things over and over . . . — to wake up, pay attention, try to face how strange, miraculous and fearful it is, every life, every day. That hurts too, waking up, finding oneself so small and vulnerable, knowing nothing. But suffering holds gifts, rich and mysterious gifts concealed in the dark folds of pain. . . .

— KATHRYN WALKER, *A Stopover in Venice*

[L]ife is an extraordinarily vast thing. And when you use the word "life," it is all the oceans and the mountains and the trees and all of human aspirations, human miseries, despairs, struggles, the immensity of it all.

— J. KRISHNAMURTI, *Krishnamurti on Education*

Preface

> Even in the midst of great pain, Lord,
> I praise you for that which is.
> — Stephen Mitchell, *A Book of Psalms*

In 2000 the blinding pain of incapacitating headaches nearly destroyed my career. The wisdom about pain, suffering, and healing that the headaches would reveal is the subject of this book. It describes how Buddhist teachings and daily meditation can empower you, the reader, to heal the suffering caused by physical and emotional pain. As the book shows, Buddhist teachings also provide a new lens for reading the Bible, yielding fresh insights into fundamental questions of birth and death, ego and enlightenment, sickness and health — insights that speak in surprisingly relevant ways to spiritual seekers and to those who want to heal themselves. My goal in writing this book is to inspire you to reexamine your experiences with suffering and pain and eventually to embrace your life with equanimity, gratitude, and joy.

The blinding pain blinded me to the liberating, simple truth that is the heart of the Buddha's teaching. Pain is unavoidable, but suffering can end. A path that leads to the end of suffering is mindfulness, which is cultivated by meditation. This book relates my experience in trying to understand the wisdom expressed in these two, short sentences. It took many years because the truth, though simple, cannot be grasped intellectually. You must live with the pain and accept the pain and breathe with the pain and breathe through the pain before you can discern the vast landscape that opens up beyond it, a landscape created by the pain itself.

This book is not about me. It is about our shared humanity, what causes suffering and what brings happiness. This book is about the wisdom of Buddhist teachings, which can change your life if you open yourself up to them. I will share this wisdom using my life as a lens, filtering my experiences with awareness, compassion, and honesty. In so doing, I will share insights that have benefited me and that I hope can therefore benefit you.

My story is easily summarized. After decades of searching I didn't see that I was lost. Then it found me. It saved me. It gave me wings that lifted me up out of the suffering caused by chronic headaches by inviting me to face the pain rather than curse the pain and try to push it away. It healed me with my wounds. It opened me up to the wisdom of my own body, bestowing on me, but only when I was ready, two radical insights. The truth is in my pain. The truth is in my face.

What saved me from drowning in the whirlpool of my former existence was the net of Buddhist insight and wisdom. These teachings lay out a systematic path to alleviate suffering, bring inner peace, and awaken the innate wisdom that sleeps within us. While this claim might seem far-fetched, in my experience it is absolutely true. My experience is based not on detached, intellectual curiosity, but on chronic headaches, debilitating, incapacitating headaches that could flare up without warning in the middle of my face. A phone call, a careless remark, a careful remark, missing an elevator, being followed too closely by another car: anything could trigger them and everything did.

When the headaches first erupted in February 2000, I suffered from the pain and even more from my outrage over the pain. What did I do to deserve this? With one exception, all the doctors I consulted ranged from being clueless to disastrous. The many pills they prescribed were ineffective and even dangerous as they changed my personality and sucked up all my intellectual and emotional energy.

Desperate, unable to find relief from medication, I turned to meditation. As this book describes, the meditation has helped me deal with the headaches much more effectively than I ever dreamed. It has taught me not to react. It has taught me to see. Healing me with my wounds, meditation has blossomed from a practical technique for dealing with headaches into an all-encompassing approach to my life. As I have learned, so can you also learn.

If like me you suffer from chronic pain, then you are not alone. In an article in *Time Magazine* Claudia Wallis points out that approximately one-sixth of the US population suffers from chronic or recurrent pain, and of these about half find no good solution. If you are one of these people, then perhaps aspects of my experience will be familiar to you. Perhaps you are now in the place where I was when the headaches first erupted. If so, then there is hope because, as my story shows, in the dark folds of pain healing can bloom.

However, if you are not a chronic-pain sufferer, then perhaps the descriptions of my suffering will strike you as the yammering of an obsessive mind. There are numerous health issues much more serious than my own.

But the Buddha (meaning "the awakened one") is subtle and wise. My suffering from pain is symptomatic of the human condition, in which the Buddha saw suffering in a much wider and deeper sense. His term was *dukkha*, which includes but goes far beyond suffering from illness and pain. The Buddha explained it in the First Noble Truth (translation by Walpola Rahula):

> The Noble Truth of suffering *(Dukkha)* is this: Birth is suffering; aging is suffering, sickness is suffering; death is suffering; sorrow and lamentation, pain, grief and despair are suffering; association with the unpleasant is suffering; dissociation from the pleasant is suffering; not to get what one wants is suffering — in brief, the five aggregates of attachment are suffering.

Dukkha is pervasive and deep. It is the uncertainty and angst arising from our sense that things are not quite right because we don't have enough and can't hold onto what we have and what we have doesn't bring lasting satisfaction and therefore we must persist acquiring and doing rather than just be. Often subtle, *dukkha* is huge, the specter that haunts us while we are asleep and while we think we are awake, always craving, always unhappy, always searching. The Buddha said that he taught one thing and only one thing: *dukkha* and the end of *dukkha*. The goal of his teachings was to expand our awareness of this fundamental aspect of our human existence, awareness leading to change, leading to peace.

Most of us suffer, whether from physical pain, emotional pain, or the *dukkha* of the human condition. What is your suffering? I have suffered, not only from headaches, but also from a complex relationship with my father, who taught me so much but never let me get close to him, and from the chaos of my graduate-school years when the Vietnam War draft gagged and blindfolded my literary soul, and from a research-level math book published in 1985, and from the "great Jewish novel" that I spent fifteen years writing but could never publish, and from having to say goodbye to my children when they grew up. All of which exploded in the headache attack of 2000. As the Buddha taught, my suffering was rooted in illusion, attachment, aversion, and ego. But I was not to see this until I faced the pain and learned from the pain and the pain woke me up.

The pain, once my brutal enemy, has become my beloved teacher, inviting me to let go and to accept. To let go of the suffering. To let go of the image of myself as a victim. Above all, to let go of the past: the complex relationship with my father, the Vietnam War draft, the 1985 math book, the great Jewish novel I couldn't publish. To accept the present moment with perfect trust.

One cannot learn how to alleviate *dukkha* before one becomes aware of it. If reading my story, the wisdom of Buddhist teachings, the wisdom of the Bible, and insights into pain, suffering, and healing helps you become more deeply aware of the *dukkha* in your life, then I will have succeeded.

Although only my name appears on the title page, I did not write this book alone. From the preconscious, Garden-of-Eden years of my youth until today, my life has been blessed by infinite richness, wisdom, and wonder, a boundless web of interdependence and love. First of all, I would like to thank my family. What my wife, Alison, has given me is so vast, yet so textured and intimate that words cannot describe it. My parents, Helen and Murray — may his memory be for a blessing — provided a safe and supportive home, in which I was raised to love learning and to love being Jewish. Alison's mother and father, Rose and Mike — may their memories be for a blessing — were my second parents, who opened up to me their home and their hearts. Our children, Melissa and Michael, are the flowers on the tree of life that Alison and I planted outside Eden, in Amherst and in Israel. Our children and their spouses, Ken and Lauren, and Melissa's and Ken's children, Noah and Lilah, are constant reminders of the love that binds us together across the generations. My brother, Ron, and his wife, Danielle, have realized their dream of living in Israel with their children and grandchildren, but I miss them very much. I am grateful to Ron for teaching me about the psychological wisdom of the Torah. Sheila and Alan, my sister-in-law and brother-in-law, have been my companions and guides for more than forty years. You are all part of me. I love you all.

    I have also been blessed by the love and support of many teachers and healers. Ted Slovin introduced me to Buddhist meditation as a way to heal suffering and alleviate pain. My rabbi, Sheila Weinberg, opened the door for me to teach the Hebrew Bible and supported me in many ways, both Jewish and Buddhist. Dr. Nagagopal Venna, my neurologist at the Massachusetts General Hospital, treated me with compassion, sensitivity, and understanding. Jean Colucci — may her memory be for a blessing — was my therapist and guide to Buddhist meditation and Buddhist wisdom. She helped me heal the suffering brought on by the headaches and helped me change my life. Joseph Goldstein and other teachers at the Insight Meditation Society in Barre, Massachusetts and Mu Soeng at the Barre Center for Buddhist Studies embodied the Buddhist wisdom that they imparted to me. Henry McKean and Srinivasa Varadhan introduced me to mathematical research at the Courant Institute of Mathematical Sciences. My passion for mathematics and literature, which had been nurtured by my father, was ignited at Harvard. David Ragozin was my first teacher of higher mathematics, Arthur Jaffe taught me mathematical physics, and Christa Saas introduced me to the wondrous landscape of German literature and the poetry of Rilke.

I have benefited greatly from three people who helped me with this book. Bob Schwartz's careful reading led to a much more focused text. Brian Burrell guided me through every step of the process of finding a publisher and was a constant support. Shmuel Bolozky helped me transliterate the Hebrew in the Hebrew Bible.

I am grateful to my colleagues in the Department of Mathematics and Statistics and in the Department of Judaic and Near Eastern Studies at the University of Massachusetts Amherst. They have provided me with the perfect atmosphere to grow both intellectually and spiritually. The most meaningful interactions of my mathematical career have been with the many collaborators and the many students — especially the graduate students who obtained Ph.D.'s under my direction — whom I have had the good fortune to meet and work with.

I would like to express my deep gratitude to Michael, my son, who grasps the Buddhist teachings intuitively. He read several versions of this book, and his suggestions improved it greatly. May the teachings continue to enlighten him as he and they have enlightened me.

It is a blessing to be alive. It is a blessing to have opened myself up to the wisdom of the pain. I hope that by reading this book, you too will understand how pain can become your best teacher.

Introduction

> The prince born twenty-five hundred years ago who became the historical Buddha ["the awakened one"] was the only founder of a major world religion who claimed to be neither a god nor a messenger of a god. When asked once just what he was, he replied simply, "I am awake."
>
> — Jean Smith, *Radiant Mind: Essential Buddhist Teachings and Texts*

BUDDHIST MEDITATION HAS changed my life. It can also change yours. I started on the path of falling in love and raising a family, discovering mathematics and literature, Israel and the Bible. But it became the path of achievement, success, and overreaching, which brought upon me the curse of chronic, incapacitating headaches. When Buddhist meditation enabled me to face the pain, the suffering ceased and the curse became a blessing, blossoming, after years of anger and struggle, into acceptance and peace.

What is your path?

Whatever path you are following, you can learn from mine because my story is a variation on a common theme. Blessed with first-rate Western educations and enjoying successful careers, about wisdom we learn nothing until it is almost too late. Then we must learn wisdom the hard way, the Buddha's way of suffering and the end of suffering. As I learned, so can you learn.

In order to help you discover your path, this book is a web interwoven with many strands: meditation, Buddhist teachings, spiritual healing, inspiration, self-help, the interpretive power of the Bible. Each strand enriches and supports the others while illuminating a main theme: how Buddhist teachings can give us the wings that will lift us out of the maelstrom of an unaware life in which we focus on ego and suffer. Most of us suffer, whether from physical pain, emotional pain, or the dissatisfaction and sense of lack that, as the Buddha taught, is pervasive in our lives. By sharing Buddhist teachings and insights into pain, suffering, and healing, I hope that you will gain greater awareness into your own suffering, awareness leading to change, leading to peace.

If you suffer from pain and turn onto the path of meditation, then pain will become your best teacher. Here is what it can teach you:

- Pain is inevitable, but suffering is optional. Meditation can help you heal suffering and alleviate pain.

- By quieting the mind, meditation allows the body's natural healing powers to flourish.

- Meditation can help you heal suffering by enabling you to slow down, to be in the moment, and to pay attention, with a light touch and without judgment, to what is pleasant, unpleasant, and neutral.

- Everything in your life is interconnected.

- Accept your pain. Embrace it. It's an integral part of your life. Open yourself up to the wisdom of your pain. That wisdom can be inexhaustible if you let it unfold.

- By accepting and embracing your pain, you may eventually come to love it. Cursing your pain, hating it, pushing it away create duality and more suffering.

- Pain wants to be a verb, not a noun, an energy flow, not a thick, brick wall. Relax. Open up. Observe it changing and flowing, surging and vanishing.

- No matter how bad your pain is, it could always be worse. Gratitude and compassion are two of its fruits.

If you turn onto the path of meditation, then you will discover a new way of being as meditation grows from a practical technique for dealing with pain into an all-encompassing approach to your life. It will change the way you process all your interactions with the world around you and the world within you. I, the permanent, rigid ego, transformed into "I," a permeable and flexible label. Less solidity, more flow. Less grasping, more letting be and letting go.

You wake up in the morning or in the middle of the night when pain makes sleep difficult. Medication has not been helping, so you have turned to meditation. You start by closing your eyes and surveying the landscape. Perhaps the pain disappears — cumulus clouds drifting across a deep, blue sky. Perhaps it does not — an emptiness in the heart, a burning or stabbing in the forehead or pinching pressure in the nose, pain precisely where you want to focus on your breath. Whatever landscape appears, you breathe through the quiet or through the pain and enter a refuge of awareness, being, and direct experience past all the concepts of good, bad, pain, suffering. The solid chunk of sensation when your eyes are open flows when your eyes are closed, flowing and rolling, waxing and waning, ocean waves lapping the shores of your inner face as you breathe through the waves, swimming, you're swimming, you're meditating. Pain, a frozen Berlin wall guarded by demons, melts into a pulsing or a burning or a throbbing or a breathing. Even when your eyes are open, you learn not to label and not to judge. The rock-hard concept of pain dissolves into an energy flow, here today, gone tomorrow, back the day after. Greetings, honored teacher. What will you teach me today? When the flow threatens to solidify, you verbify it by laughing.

If you have meditated, then perhaps you have had these experiences. They have been my experiences, giving rise to insights that I would like to share in the context of my life. I start with a summer day in my youth, July 27, 1963. While attending Alison Feinberg's sweet sixteen party, I was so captivated by her smile that I immediately fell in love with her. I went on to Harvard, Alison and I got married, we moved to New Jersey, I worked at Bell Labs to escape the Vietnam War draft, and I earned a Ph.D. in mathematics at NYU. I taught at Northwestern University, our daughter Melissa was born, then our son Michael. By this time we had gone back East, where I was teaching at the University of Massachusetts Amherst and was leading the stressed-out life of husband, father, son, teacher, and hyper-achieving, hyper-driven mathematics researcher, always aiming for more and always unsatisfied.

My family could have been enough for me. If at the time I had tried to articulate it, I might have said that I was on a quest for fulfillment beyond what I thought my family could provide. As the Buddha taught 2,500 years ago and as I would later find out, that quest was doomed from the start. The details of your life are surely different, but perhaps my story resonates with you.

For years I had been searching, my ego butting into me wherever I turned. Since my youth, I looked to mathematics, but the truth wasn't there. Since my youth, I looked to literature, but the truth wasn't there. As an adult, I looked to Israel, but the truth wasn't there. After returning from Israel, I looked to the Hebrew Bible. Perhaps the truth was there, but I could not find it. I also looked to Jewish practice: eating only kosher food, saying the daily prayers, observing the Sabbath. But those activities so disrupted my family that I dropped them.

For me today, the truth is not in mathematics and not in books and not in ego and not in heaven and not beyond the sea. It is not hidden from me, nor is it far off. I learned the truth by facing my headaches, listening to them, and learning from them. As Buddhist meditation would eventually help me understand, the truth is in my pain. The truth is in my face. This book is a record of my trying to penetrate the paradox of these insights, which would lead to my healing. What I had thought for years was the problem is actually the solution.

The blessings continue to blossom. Meditation has opened my eyes to the awareness that the pain is not my deadly enemy, but my life-enhancing teacher. Enriched by this awareness, I have also found in Buddhist teachings a key to synthesize what for years were the disparate elements out of which I have built my intellectual life — mathematics, literature, and the Hebrew Bible. In explaining this synthesis, I will share the spirituality of mathematics and Buddhist truths embedded in the Hebrew

Bible, which a Buddhist reading sensitive to the original language of the Bible reveals.

Franz Kafka's parable, "The Leopards in the Temple," describes the process that my awakening has followed. "Leopards break into the temple and drink to the dregs what is in the sacrificial pitchers; this is repeated over and over again; finally it can be calculated in advance, and it becomes a part of the ceremony."

The headaches erupted in 2000. They were a pack of leopards that broke into my temple and drank to the dregs what I had once worshipped as my ego-accomplishments, demolishing the conceptual lens of achievement and success through which I had interpreted my life. I was fortunate to have found in Buddhist meditation a new way of living that could accommodate to the headache chaos. It finally enabled me to see that what I had once worshipped as my ego-accomplishments were as empty of inherent existence and solid, substantial reality as a rainbow, an echo, a dream, the reflection of the moon in water, the concept of pain, my next breath.

Kafka's parable about the leopards is related to a major theme of this book: the connection between conceptual thinking and paradigms or conceptual lenses. A paradigm is a set of assumptions, values, meanings, and self-images representing a way of interpreting experiences and life. As the cognitive linguist George Lakoff observes, the fundamental role of conceptual lenses in structuring our view of reality is a basic tenet of cognitive science:

> We have learned that there are certain mechanisms of thought that structure our reality. What this means is that you don't see reality as it is. That's impossible from the point of view of cognitive science. You are always imposing a structure

on reality; there's no way you could do otherwise given the nature of your brain and body.

    Kafka's leopards break into the temple when an event occurs or a discovery is made that cannot be explained by the accepted paradigm. One must adapt either by altering the accepted paradigm or, if the event or discovery is too radical, by adopting a new paradigm. "Finally it can be calculated in advance, and it becomes a part of the ceremony." The paradigm shifts, the event or discovery fits into the new scheme, a different conceptual universe is born, and the leopards break into the temple again.

    When you view a rainbow, what do you see? The answer reflects the conceptual lens you are using. The physicist sees an arc of colors that appears in the sky as a result of the dispersion of sunlight in drops of mist or rain. To lovers the rainbow is a symbol of their passion; Orthodox Jews see in it a symbol of God's covenant to Noah after the flood; and movie buffs think of the better place "somewhere over the rainbow" of which Dorothy dreams in *The Wizard of Oz*. The spiritual seeker whispers "Wow," and the complainer is reminded of how rain always ruins his picnics. Who is correct? Everyone and no one.

    As with a rainbow, so with all our experiences. Without a conceptual lens, we cannot process the infinite complexity of the universe, which includes the infinite complexity of our lives and minds. The paradox, or perhaps the tragedy of the human condition, is that whatever lens we use — the lens of cognitive science, physics, or religion, the lens of romance or Hollywood entertainment — by necessity it imposes a judgment concerning expected behavior, and it excludes many other lenses. Furthermore, the sharper a lens's focus, the more it excludes. As a result, the always changing, always flowing dance of reality cannot be captured by any single conceptual lens. Leopards keep breaking into the temple because the ultimate truth is that there is no ultimate truth.

In this book we will explore pain and suffering, healing and happiness, ego and enlightenment through several conceptual lenses. These include the Hebrew Bible in translation, the radically different conceptual lens of the Hebrew Bible in its original language, and Buddhist teachings, which in this context play a fundamental role. They provide the broadest framework for understanding conceptual lenses because they go to the root, showing us how to transcend all conceptual lenses via a systematic path that alleviates suffering, brings inner peace, and awakens the innate wisdom that sleeps within us.

In order to justify this claim about Buddhist teachings, I next summarize the Buddha's insights on conceptual thinking. They will lead us to the Four Noble Truths, the heart of his diagnosis of human suffering and the end of suffering. Together with other Buddhist teachings that I was able to integrate into my life through the practice of meditation, the Four Noble Truths led to my healing. In discussing these teachings in the context of my experiences, I hope to inspire you to explore them and ultimately to benefit from them in the same profound way that I have.

By their very nature, conceptual lenses inevitably lead to limited vision. Buying into a single lens, without the awareness that it is only a lens, is what the Buddha called attachment to views. In his book, *Old Path, White Clouds: Walking in the Footsteps of the Buddha*, Thich Nhat Hanh discusses why "attachment to views is the greatest impediment to the spiritual path. . . . Thinking that we already possess the truth, we will be unable to open our minds to receive the truth, even if truth comes knocking at our door." Attachment to views inevitably causes suffering in the sense of the Buddha's term *dukkha,* which includes not only suffering from physical pain, mental anguish, and grief but also much more. Christopher W. Gowans explains that suffering is too narrow a translation to convey the broad range of implications that *dukkha* conveys:

> For example, it sometimes implies such things as disappointment, frustration, anxiety, discontentment, dissatisfaction, lack of fulfillment, falling short of perfection, and the absence of ease. In addition, the meaning of *"dukkha"* is broad enough that it might be interpreted as encompassing . . . a sense of finitude, melancholy, alienation, and *angst.* . . . *Dukkha* . . . is perhaps most usefully thought of as the failure to fully achieve an ideal of happiness we all implicitly seek. . . .

In the Fire Sermon the Buddha gave one of his strongest images, analogizing the *dukkha* that arises from conceptual thinking to a raging fire (translation by Thanissaro Bhikkhu):

> The intellect is aflame. Ideas are aflame. Consciousness at the intellect is aflame. Contact at the intellect is aflame. And whatever there is that arises in dependence on contact at the intellect — experienced as pleasure, pain or neither-pleasure-nor-pain — that too is aflame. Aflame with what? Aflame with the fire of passion, the fire of aversion, the fire of delusion. Aflame, I say, with birth, aging and death, with sorrows, lamentations, pains, distresses, and despairs.

Through conceptual lenses, the outer eye learns how to see, but seeing without awareness inevitably brings *dukkha*. Meditation helps extinguish the raging fire. The inner eye learns wisdom, we become aware of whatever conceptual lens we are wearing, and ultimately we transcend all lenses, viewing reality as it is. Enlightenment, the Buddha called this. Nirvana. Thich Nhat Hanh elucidates this term in his book, *Understanding Our Mind*:

> Nirvana means stability, freedom, and the cessation of the cycle of suffering. Enlightenment does not come from outside; it is not something we are given, even by a Buddha. The seed of enlightenment is already within our consciousness. This is our Buddha nature — the inherent quality of enlightened mind that we all possess, and which needs only to be nurtured.

The Buddha formulated his insights into *dukkha* in the Four Noble Truths. He enunciated them in his first discourse after meditating under the Bodhi tree and attaining enlightenment, and they remained the main focus of his forty-five years of teaching. These in brief are the Four Noble Truths:

1. There is suffering.
2. Suffering originates in attachment: attachment to desire, to craving for sense pleasures, to one's own views, to the belief in I and self.
3. Suffering can end and peace can be experienced.
4. The way that leads to the end of suffering and to experiencing peace is the path of being mindful, of seeing reality as it is, not through the conceptual lens of I and

self. This way is the Noble Eightfold Path comprising right understanding, right intention, right speech, right action, right livelihood, right effort, right mindfulness, and right concentration. The last three qualities are cultivated by practicing meditation.

In our ignorance we seek happiness by attachment to desire, to craving for sense pleasures, to one's own views, to the belief in I and self. But this is doomed because it contradicts the nature of reality. Transient, continually flowing, empty of any solid, inherent existence, reality is governed by the universal law of impermanence and change. Everything is changing on every level all the time, and nothing stays fixed, not only material possessions but also bodies, mental states, relationships, experiences, entire civilizations and cultures. Refusing to accept this universal truth, we grasp at the impermanent, hoping that it will stay fixed, and when it inevitably does not, we suffer. We can overcome suffering and become truly happy not by attachment to what must pass, but by accepting the universal law of impermanence and change as the guiding principle of our lives.

This book examines the Four Noble Truths through the conceptual lenses of chronic pain, meditation, the Hebrew Bible, and mathematics. What are your lenses? Through them, let the truth of the Four Noble Truths permeate your life.

1. I suffered.

2. I suffered because I craved recognition and fame through mathematics and other intellectual pursuits and because I craved to get rid of the pain. Not understanding that pain is a concept, I congealed it into a solid, substantial reality and then suffered from that solidification.

3. I learned that suffering could end and peace could be experienced.

4. Meditation showed me the path by revealing the truth of the pain: the pain is impermanent, continually flowing and changing, empty of any solid, substantial reality. Facing the truth that is in my face, I let go of the pain, let go of the past, let go of the ego, and finally woke up.

A fly caught in a windowless room, we solidify our pain into a windowpane against which we keep smashing our faces. The pain intensifies; the pane grows thicker. Panic. We are trapped. No, we're not. The pane of pain is a mirror in which we see that the door has been open all the time. Look again. The pane of pain is empty space, and we can fly right through.

There is no pain. There is no pane. There is no solidity, certainty, or permanence. There is only change and empty space. Now is all we have.

Listen to the Buddha. When asked why his disciples were so radiant, he gave the following answer, recorded by David Loy in his book, *Lack and Transcendence*:

> "They do not repent of the past, nor do they brood over the future. They live in the present. Therefore they are radiant. By brooding over the future and repenting the past, fools dry up like green reeds cut down [in the sun]."

The past and the future are merely conceptual abstractions. Opening to the present is the most precious present we can give ourselves. Meditation teaches us how.

These are the insights I have learned and want to share with you. I did not learn them from books. I learned them through suffering and overcoming suffering. I learned them by opening up to the present and forgiving myself for the past.

In this spirit of forgiveness, I examine some of my lives, lives that I have let go of but that illuminate the roots of the headaches and the healing. Growing up in a Jewish area of Boston; meeting Alison, my wife, lover, and best friend; double-majoring in mathematics and German literature at Harvard; having to abort my post-Harvard plans because of the Vietnam War draft; working on my Ph.D.; surviving the first headache attack of 1980; discovering Israel and my Jewish soul in 1982; publishing my first math book in 1985; not publishing the "great Jewish novel," on which I labored for fifteen years; publishing a second math book in 1997 that I wrote with Paul Dupuis; experiencing the poetry of Emily Dickinson; teaching courses on the Hebrew Bible and Franz Kafka; publishing articles on the Hebrew Bible, literature, and the Holocaust; almost not surviving the headache earthquake of 2000.

That earthquake was a defining event on my journey of awakening. The injustice of it all, to be zapped by headaches in the prime of my life. "Why me?" I screamed. "Why now?" How I suffered from the pain and how I doubly suffered from my utter inability to figure out the pain and how I triply suffered from the many doctors who pumped me with pills and were deaf to my anguish, each doctor issuing his own diagnosis or no diagnosis but never really listening to me. Have you also suffered in this way?

Then I met Jean Colucci, a clinician who based her therapy on Buddhist principles. Under her guidance I began to meditate daily, and this in turn brought me to a meditation retreat. There, on August 5, 2003, through no effort of my own, an insight emerged from out of nowhere: the truth is in my pain. It was a manifestation of the innate wisdom that the Buddhists call Buddha nature and that we all possess. My suffering blossomed into healing when I opened myself up to Buddhist teachings and allowed this insight about my pain to guide me. I finally woke up from the deep sleep of duality and illusion in which I was unable to see that the pain is my honored teacher.

In this book I offer the inner experience of that awakening. With a joy of insight unmediated by any conceptual lens, I finally understood that the truth about my pain is in my face. That truth continues to resonate until today. It wrote this book.

Thus some of the lives of Richard S. Ellis, a comforting label that gives the illusion of a fixed, stable identity. These lives are transient, but the wisdom that has nourished them is real. It is the wisdom of Buddhist teachings, made accessible through the headache pain. It is also the wisdom that the Bible reveals when read with a sensitivity to the original Hebrew, to which a gentle introduction will be given. In so reading the Bible, especially the narratives, one experiences a fertile ambiguity, a fluidity of language, theme, and character pregnant with possibilities and unavailable in any translation. As we become aware of the openendedness, multiple interpretability, and vast reach of the original Hebrew, we are inspired to face our lives with the same awareness of interdependence and infinite possibilities. With practice, we begin to experience life as a flow in which we swim, not as a problem that we must solve. This is one of the Hebrew Bible's great lessons. As we will see when we explore several narratives, it speaks a Buddhist language that goes beyond words and concepts.

Because the Hebrew Bible receives much attention in this book, I would like to explain this and related terms. The Hebrew

Bible has three parts: the Five Books of Moses, the Prophets, and the Writings. The Five Books of Moses, which in Hebrew is called the Torah, comprise Genesis, Exodus, Leviticus, Numbers, and Deuteronomy. The Torah is the primary text of Judaism. It is read from a handwritten Torah scroll during Shabbat (Saturday) morning services in the synagogue. In this book the word "Torah" is also used in a second, more general sense. It is a dynamic term referring to all the teachings of Judaism, including the Hebrew Bible, as well as all commentaries and interpretations, including those in chapters 4–6 of this book and those that you contribute. In this more general sense, "Torah" is the closest word in Jewish spirituality to the Sanskrit word "Dharma," the body of teachings expounded by the Buddha and by all those inspired by the Buddha.

As I will describe in the next chapter, the Hebrew Bible discovered me in Israel. That book is my passion, but not the God who commanded Abraham to sacrifice his son Isaac, through whom Abraham had been promised that he would be a great and mighty nation. Instead, I embrace the God who played with Adam in the Garden of Eden and who argued with Abraham over the fate of the inhabitants of Sodom and Gomorrah. That is how we will read the Bible: by playing with the text as God played with Adam, by arguing with the text as Abraham argued with God.

The prosaic details and apparently routine experiences of daily life are the fertile soil in which deep insights about happiness, suffering, and healing germinate. These insights both are nourished by Buddhist teachings and elucidate these teachings when the experiences of daily life are examined with awareness, compassion, and honesty. Similarly, the apparently prosaic, all too familiar text of the Bible is the fertile soil in which deep insights about birth and death, ego and enlightenment, sickness and health germinate. These insights both are nourished by Buddhist teachings and elucidate these teachings when the Bible is read with a sensitivity to the Hebrew original.

We start with Jacob, whose story is about awareness, transformation, and acceptance. He is the quintessential Jewish hero who prevailed by his wit and his guile. Then he discovered, as I did, a new way of being, based not on achievement and control, but on insight and love. We also examine through a Buddhist lens the stories of creation and the Garden of Eden, which resonate with Buddhist teachings: the genesis of conceptual thinking, the flowering of self-consciousness, the birth of the ego-self, and the possibility of enlightenment. Finally we look at the Book of Job. Of all the books of the Bible it speaks the most eloquently about suffering, the search for justification, and spiritual growth. When pain afflicts us, we often act like Job, demanding explanations for our suffering and trying to rationalize it. But this doesn't bring peace. We will find peace when our inner voice of wisdom — our Buddha nature — reveals the truth, as Job found peace when God spoke to him from the whirlwind.

As a teacher of Biblical texts, I am aware of a great hunger for spiritual nourishment that the Bible, as it is traditionally taught, does not universally provide. The innovative readings of Bible narratives to be presented here can satisfy this hunger by yielding fruitful insights that you, the reader, could apply to change your life.

Headache pain has been my best teacher. Physical and emotional pain can also be your best teacher, becoming a path to verifying the truth of Buddhist teachings. In order to inspire you to reexamine your experiences with suffering and pain, in the next-to-last chapter I weave together personal narratives and teachings that emphasize a basic aspect of the Buddha's work.

He totally avoided metaphysical questions and focused on the practical as he pursued his goal, which was to teach people how to alleviate suffering and to find peace.

The teachings of the Buddha are profound and vast, an intricately interconnected web of insights that illuminate every facet of our experience. The Buddha also provided a path to incorporating these insights into our lives. A key component of this path is mindfulness, which is the calm and direct awareness — without judgments, concepts, or ego — of what is happening in the present moment, in our bodies, in our minds, and in the world around us. Mindfulness is cultivated by meditation. In the appendix I discuss how one might start to walk this path by learning to meditate. Brief instructions for meditation are also given.

Just as Buddhist teachings have changed my life, so they can also change yours, whether you suffer from the *dukkha* of chronic pain, the *dukkha* of emotional pain, or the *dukkha* of the human condition. In the spaciousness of that landscape that is beyond I, beyond separation, conflicts, concepts, constructs, and confusion, your innate Buddha nature will unfold if you allow it to. In his book, *The Healing Power of Mind*, Tulku Thondup describes this process:

> Living beings are Buddha in their true nature,
> But their nature is obscured by casual or sudden afflictions.
> When the afflictions are cleansed, living beings themselves are the very Buddha.
>
> Buddhahood, or enlightenment, is "no-self." It is total, everlasting, universal peace, openness, selflessness, oneness, and joy.

How can we strip away our many conceptual lenses to become aware of our Buddha nature and to experience our lives and all creation with love, gratitude, and wonder? This book is a meditation on that question, which goes to the heart of the Buddha's teachings and to the heart of everyone's awakening. May the meditation on this question also help you discover the path to a more tranquil and fulfilling life, in which your suffering is transformed into peace.

1
Letting Go of the Past

> The past is over: Forgiveness means giving
> up all hope of a better past.
> — Jack Kornfeld, *The Art of Forgiveness,
> Lovingkindness, and Peace*

How shall one write about the past when one has let it go?

Letting go of the past does not mean throwing it away. Letting go means letting be. It means accepting all the pain of all our years. We have wounded ourselves. We have wounded others. We have been wounded. The past is over. We have suffered. We have caused ourselves to suffer. We have caused others to suffer. The past is over. We have achieved. We haven't achieved enough. Our craving for fame has harmed others and ourselves. The past is over. We have loved. We have not loved enough. We have been loved by an infinite love. The past is over. Letting go means accepting, deeply and without conditions, that we are human.

Letting go of the past means focusing, in the present book, on the headaches and the healing. It means letting go of all the accomplishments: graduate of Harvard in mathematics and German literature; Professor of Mathematics; Adjunct Professor of Judaic Studies; mathematician with a theorem named after me; self-taught Bible exegete and teacher; author of high-level math books, articles on literature, and a novel I couldn't publish. Above all, letting go of the past means forgiving ourselves for having acted out of fear, anger, and confusion. Jack Kornfeld was a co-founder of the Insight Meditation Society in Barre, Massachusetts, where I experienced the truth about my pain in August 2003. A central theme of his book, *The Art of Forgiveness, Lovingkindness, and Peace*, and a central theme of my journey are that "[f]orgiveness is the necessary ground for any healing":

> Finding a way to extend forgiveness to ourselves is one of our most essential tasks. Just as others have been caught in suffering, so have we. If we look honestly at our lives, we can see the sorrows and pain that have led to our own wrongdoing. In this we can finally extend forgiveness to ourselves; we can hold the pain we have caused in compassion. Without such mercy, we will live our own life in exile.

In this spirit of forgiveness I start every meditation session by repeating these comforting words, which I learned at a retreat in 2006 from Mark Coleman, one of the retreat leaders:

> In whatever ways I may have harmed myself, knowingly or unknowingly, through my words,

speech, or action, I offer myself forgiveness, as much as I am able to in this moment.

In whatever ways I may have harmed others, knowingly or unknowingly, through my words, speech, or action, I ask them for forgiveness, as much as I am able to in this moment.

In whatever ways others may have harmed me, knowingly or unknowingly, through their words, speech, or action, I offer them forgiveness, as much as I am able to in this moment.

In this spirit of forgiveness, I now give you some of my lives, lives that I have let go of but that illuminate the roots of the headaches and the healing. The insights that the pain has taught me cannot be separated from the experiences in which the insights occurred. We are human, and being human is to experience the truth through a body and in specific places. The paradox of introspection is that by shining the light of awareness on what is uniquely our own, we address the universal.

My journey of awakening began on July 27, 1963. While attending Alison Feinberg's sweet sixteen party, I saw Alison smile. In a moment of pure consciousness I couldn't articulate then, her soft, gentle smile became a laser light piercing the shell that swathed my adolescent soul, and I immediately fell in love with her. The experience pointed to a new way of being, based on love, not on achievement, a way of being I never knew existed. It spoke a wordless language I would not be able to understand for many years. Never before had I experienced anything so beautiful. That smile still moves me today.

My high school was Boston Latin School. In 1965 I graduated second in the class of 295 students, missing out on first place by a fraction of a percentage point caused by one grade of 75% in senior physics. At the time, my missing out on first place was the only blemish in the otherwise flawless, academic tapestry of my unaware life. My parents and I had become emotionally distant; I would not have a meaningful conversation with my brother Ron until we were adults; and I had tried to fill the emotional void of my adolescence by falling in love with two different girlfriends before I met Alison. But none of this registered.

I was blinded to the truth by the white light of what I discovered at Boston Latin School to be my life's calling: to excel and to achieve. It was a calling that became a curse and then a blessing because facing the curse years later through the lens of facial pain forced me to change. How easily the string of A's came to me and how proud I was of them, unprepared for the suffering that this would eventually bring upon me.

At Harvard, academic success but spiritual hollowness: a double major in mathematics and German literature; an honors thesis on Schrödinger Hamiltonians in quantum mechanics and an honors thesis on Apollo and the Buddha in the *New Poems* of Rainer Maria Rilke. How ironic that I wrote about the Buddha. His wisdom, filtered through Rilke's poetry, spoke to me even in my youth when I was so unaware.

Under Rilke's inspiration, I filled notebooks with my own poetry. I experienced my soul bifurcate into Apollo versus the Buddha, mathematics versus literature, analytic thinking versus poetry, precision versus spirituality — dualities expressed by me in the coda of a sonnet that I published in a Harvard literary journal:

> Birth under Taurus: two cool blue skies
> that mirror the earth of these moody eyes.

When I graduated from Harvard, I stood like Moses on the border of a promised land I could not enter, this one a landscape of literary studies in Germany and advanced mathematics at Princeton, my path blocked not by God, but by the Vietnam War draft.

Instead of spending a year studying literature in Heidelberg and then moving on to graduate study at Princeton, I reluctantly accepted a draft-deferred job at Bell Laboratories. It kept me out of the army but gagged and blindfolded my newly emergent poetic soul. The job was extremely generous. In exchange for working part-time, I received a salary and the opportunity to obtain my Ph.D. at the Courant Institute of Mathematical Sciences at New York University, which Bell Labs fully financed.

The Courant Institute of Mathematical Sciences had been established by Richard Courant after World War II as a reincarnation of the Mathematics Institute at the University of Göttingen, the world's greatest concentration of mathematical genius until the Nazis destroyed it. Initially staffed with many Jewish émigré mathematicians from Germany, the Courant Institute was, and continues to be, one of the premier centers of applied mathematics in the world. For this budding, yet sensitive, young mathematician who probably would have found Princeton too aggressive and competitive, it provided a comfortable, supporting atmosphere.

Being able to attend the Courant Institute was the hidden blessing of the Vietnam War draft because it allowed my life's path to intersect that of Henry McKean. As my Ph.D. advisor, Henry is in the first rank of all the benefactors who have blessed me with their knowledge, insight, and love. The afternoon we spent together was the high point of every week. Inhaling inspiration through an unfiltered Camel, Henry was a magician. He always came up with a new approach to a problem whenever he got stuck, teaching me that there is always another way. Henry was my hero, the only benevolent father-figure in my life, and I have revered him ever since.

My weekly afternoon with Henry McKean was the counterbalance to the days I had to spend at Bell Labs, which I loathed. So much luckier than almost all of my friends, I remained miserable from the moment I first entered the drab Bell Labs building in Whippany, New Jersey until I was liberated three years later by a draft-lottery number of 130, which was 10 above the cutoff. Although I was jubilant, no trumpets sounded as I walked to my car for the final time in the Bell Labs parking lot and drove off, about to start a new life in Evanston, Illinois, where I had accepted a tenure-track position at Northwestern University.

Meanwhile, my Jewish soul had atrophied. Having grown up in an Orthodox family in a Jewish area of Boston, I quit Hebrew school right after my bar mitzvah and ceased having any involvement with the ancestral religion at all. Through my years at Harvard and NYU and our first years of marriage, I rejected it as a secret society of old men practicing meaningless rituals that had no bearing on my heart and on my mind. Mathematics and literature ignited my soul. The Hebrew Bible was a locked book.

Only through the Holocaust did I remain passionately, though negatively, committed to Judaism. It started while I was at Harvard with movies, diaries, personal testimonies, historical analyses, and photographs, and I couldn't get enough. *The Rise and Fall of the Third Reich* by William L. Shirer became my Bible. My bookshelves bulging with books about the Holocaust, it was natural that my novel would feature a partisan who murdered Nazis in the woods near Vilna.

In 1975 I took a position at the University of Massachusetts Amherst because Alison and I wanted to be closer to our families in Boston. My teaching and research went so well that I was given early tenure and promotion. But I was working too hard — too many papers, too many trips. Then my father contracted colon cancer, which he kept a secret from everyone except my mother, causing both of them to suffer — the malodor emanating from the colostomy bag was a constant embarrassment for them both — and when I tried to help by recommending therapy, my father became so angry that he stopped talking with me for half a year. Then Michael was born, a non-sleeper who gave us two years of nights with interrupted sleep.

In March 1980 vicious tension headaches attacked the top of my head, which felt as if it were being sliced open with a rusty hacksaw. I was saved by Ted Slovin, a therapist who taught me relaxation techniques and gave me my first lessons in Buddhist meditation. How lucky I was to find him. Because Ted's therapy was so effective, I began to explore intellectually the wisdom of the Buddhist tradition, finding in it the clearest statement of spiritual truths that I had ever encountered. Buddhism and Judaism, I would later realize, have much in common. However, in the early 1980s the spiritual treasures of Judaism were locked away in a fortified palace swaddled in fog high on the mountain, at the base of which the clear running water of Buddhism flowed.

The Buddhism of the early 1980s was all in the head and not in the heart. Replete with knowledge but bereft of wisdom, I practiced the relaxation techniques only as long as the headaches lasted. As soon as the headaches stopped in 1981, so did the daily practice, without which the spiritual teachings dissipated like water in a holey bucket. Overwork and stress had led to the tension headaches. After the relaxation techniques had healed them, did I stop working hard, as my headaches warned that I should? I couldn't stop, and I threw myself into the new project of a research-level math book.

To my surprise, in the midst of all the turmoil, my Jewish soul was slowly awakening. Reluctantly I let my wife convince me to join a synagogue in Amherst, where I actually enjoyed the guitar-strumming cantor who played at High Holiday services and who gave me the first positive synagogue experience in my life. We began to attend Sabbath services and became interested in Israel.

This opening set the stage for an almost random event that would change our lives. At the bat mitzvah of a niece in 1981, Alison and I had a casual conversation with a friend about the wonders of Israel, where the friend's daughter lived. I had a sabbatical the next year, and on the spur of the moment Alison and I decided to spend a semester in Israel although we knew no one there. I received a fellowship that supported me during the spring semester of 1982 as a visiting professor at the Technion – Israel Institute of Technology in Haifa.

Living in that holy place a quarter of the planet away allowed me to reclaim the Jewish identity that I had abandoned after my bar mitzvah. Through our 10,000 kilometers of travel in Israel, through the deep friendships that we formed, and through our love affair with the land and the people, I made two discoveries. First, there are other paths to Judaism — cultural, literary, historical — besides the path through the synagogue, which for many American Jews is often the only path. Second, the joy of living in Israel, learning the history, and participating in the culture were the perfect counterbalance to my obsession with the Holocaust. In turn, opening myself up to my Jewish heritage would enable me eventually to teach the Bible and would open me up to the wisdom of Buddhist teachings.

Israel was also the place where in 1982 I started to write my first math book, *Entropy, Large Deviations, and Statistical Mechanics*. Mathematically, a large deviation is a random event having small probability and often significant effect; for example, being dealt a royal straight flush in a high-stakes poker game. More broadly, a large deviation is any event defying expectations: a surprise, a disaster, a miracle. We begin to see large deviations everywhere as we live our lives more openly, more meditatively, more Buddhistly. In his book of essays, *The Lives of a Cell: Notes of a Biology Watcher*, Lewis Thomas points out the most fundamental large-deviation fact of all, which everyone would claim to know but few seem to understand. This fact is the miracle of being alive, the awareness of which should "keep us all in a contented dazzlement of surprise":

> Statistically, the probability of any one of us being here is so small that you'd think the mere fact of existing would keep us all in a contented dazzlement of surprise. We are alive against the stupendous odds of genetics, infinitely outnumbered by all the alternates who might, except for luck, be in our places.

My math book focused on the theory of large deviations in probability and statistical mechanics, which uses probabilistic models to analyze physical systems consisting of large numbers of particles. The theory of large deviations has significant applications not only in probability and statistical mechanics, but also in nonlinear dynamics, statistics, information theory, engineering, and biology, in the study of turbulence, traffic flow, and financial markets, in weather prediction, medical prognosis, and the evolution of language, and in other creative outpourings of nature and the human mind. I am equally interested in the mathematical content of the theory and in its applicability to my life — a life that has been a large deviation in numerous ways, Jewish, literary, spiritual, and mathematical.

My passion for mathematics reached its zenith-nadir in 1985. In that year I published *Entropy, Large Deviations, and Statistical Mechanics*, which brought me suffering as well as recognition. The suffering came because I was obsessed with fear. It was the fear of having made a catastrophic mathematical error that would cause the book's entire conceptual structure to collapse like a house of cards. As I would later suffer from the headaches, so I suffered from the book. In both cases I congealed concepts — the concept of pain, the concept of a mathematical error — into solid, substantial realities and then suffered deeply from those solidifications.

On the inside, chaos. On the outside, recognition. To my amazement, the book that had sucked me into a psychological quagmire was received by the scientific community with accolades. Perhaps the best compliment came from my son Michael, who as an undergraduate saw my book on the shelf of a professor of computer science. "When I told him that my father was the author," Michael related, "he said that it's one of his favorite books. I'm proud of you." In addition, the book highlighted a useful theorem, which, to my total surprise, came to be called the Gärtner-Ellis Theorem (Jürgen Gärtner is a German mathematician whose work I generalized).

My realization of how all the Jewish, literary, spiritual, and mathematical large deviations have impacted me has opened up a panoramic vista of insight. My life is a large deviation surrounded by boundless, unknowable mystery and infused with miracles, and the headaches are a symbol of that mystery. However, when I wrote the math book, I lost sight of the mystery of creation and the miracle of my existence. My world contracted into the pile of papers out of which the isolated I of my ego was struggling to build a monument to my intellect. The suffering that the book brought upon me was not a large deviation but the inevitable consequence of the constricted perspective nourishing the illusions under which I was living. "Suffering follows an evil thought," said the Buddha, "as the wheels of the cart follow the oxen that draw it" (translation by Eknath Easwaran).

What about the catastrophic errors in my book that I had obsessed over? Mathematically there were none, but I would not know that until well after the book had been published. There turns out to have been one embarrassing bibliographic error. Unintentionally I had shortchanged Jürgen Gärtner's contribution to the Gärtner-Ellis Theorem because I had misunderstood it.

The depth of my suffering from the book mirrors the amplitude of my love of mathematics, which I cherish because it is a spiritual undertaking akin to meditation. Even when much of my life was shrouded in illusion and confusion, mathematics allowed me to see clearly. This clarity of vision is one of its greatest gifts. Two deep theorems, Cantor's theorem on the existence of an infinite hierarchy of ever expanding infinities and Gödel's Incompleteness Theorem on the self-consistency of mathematical theories, show that mathematics is an inexhaustible, infinitely creative source of freedom and truth. The subject is all the more remarkable because this logical structure built out of symbols and concepts is illogically and extravagantly effective in giving access to the most profound secrets of the physical universe.

In the aftermath of the math book, the suffering I had brought upon myself was foremost in my mind. In order to recover, I made a six-month pilgrimage to Jerusalem with my family in 1986. While we were living there, one of the most profound, large-deviation events of my life unfolded. A cousin from the US visited us in Jerusalem and told us that a branch of my family was living in Netanya, about an hour from Jerusalem by car. That discovery closed a circle that had been broken in Parczew, Poland sixty-three years earlier. In 1923, when my grandparents and my mother, then five months old, immigrated to the US, my grandfather's brother Shulem was unable to join them. His identification papers had been taken by a cousin in order to avoid being drafted into the Polish army. Instead, Shulem immigrated to Argentina, coming to Israel with his son Yosef, my Israeli cousin, in 1952.

The story of my family has made me understand, with a visceral force, the basic Buddhist teaching about the contingency of human existence. An almost random chain of events has brought me here, to Amherst, Massachusetts via Parczew, Boston, Whippany, Evanston, Haifa, and Jerusalem, and didn't bring me to Russia or Argentina, and my mother and I were not condemned to the oblivion that swallowed up all the members of my extended family who didn't get out of Europe in time, including all eight sisters and brothers of the mother of my Israeli cousin. The eight siblings were gassed at Treblinka.

The awareness of the contingency of my existence makes me overflow with gratitude. O precious human life. I am breathing. I am loving. I am alive. Having been born, I used this gift to go to Israel. Being there opened up so much for me. Meeting an unknown branch of my family, through whom I was connected to the ancestral homeland. Living the rhythms of the Jewish week and the Jewish year. Reading James A. Michener's *The Source*, the inspirational epic of the land of Israel that made me feel, in my gut, what it means to be a Jew. Traveling through the land and seeing the Bible come alive as it discovered me: in the cave of Elijah in Haifa; in Jaffa, from which the prophet Jonah sailed; in Beersheva, from which Abraham set out for Jerusalem to fulfill God's monstrous command to sacrifice his son in chapter 22 of Genesis; and especially in Jerusalem, the place of pilgrimage ever since the time of Abraham, the illogical city that has thrived on the edge of the Judean Desert at the boundary of the Western world.

Living in Israel also opened me up to Jewish spirituality. This, in turn, allowed the teachings of the Buddha to blossom in my heart, saving me from drowning in the headache maelstrom of 2000.

Discovering my Israeli cousins while living in Jerusalem inspired a novel in which I tried to explore the suffering brought on by the math book, hoping thereby to release myself from it. I spent fifteen years writing and revising *Blessings from the Dead*, my great Jewish novel of Jerusalem, the Holocaust, mathematics, and Bible codes. Rather than being cathartic, the novel brought more suffering because publishing it became my primary goal and the goal remained beyond reach. Again Buddhist teachings opened my eyes, enabling me to transform the non-publishing from a curse into another blessing when I realized that the fifteen years of labor on the novel had helped me learn how to write. This insight was a gift from a 2003 lecture by Daniel Goleman on Buddhism and cognitive science.

I now understand that publishing the math book and not publishing the novel led me large-deviationally onto a path on which I can finally articulate the suffering and the wisdom that the two books brought me. And it all had its roots in Israel. There, in 1982 I began work on the math book to be published three years later. The psychological issues uncovered by the math book, coupled with the discovery of my Israeli cousins, made writing the novel a necessity. In turn, not being able to publish the novel was one of many challenges that culminated in the headache attack eighteen years later, a crisis from which the present book grew. Israel, the land of the book, was the place where my math book was conceived and its novelistic daughter and its Buddhist-Jewish granddaughter that you are now reading.

What happened to me in Israel was miraculous. There I discovered my Jewish soul. There I discovered that I could be Jewish without being observant. There the Bible discovered me. There I began work on the math book, and while living in Jerusalem, I recovered from the math book. But like Jews through the millennia, I could not stay in Israel. My home being in the Diaspora, I had to learn to carry Israel with me, and I did this as Jews through the millennia have done. I learned to carry Israel with me in the form of the great Jewish book, the one I love above all others: the Hebrew Bible.

It was all so natural, even fated. My four years in Hebrew school taught me to read Hebrew but with no understanding. Before going to Israel in 1982, I had forgotten how to count to ten. Both in Israel and later at home, I studied Hebrew and learned to speak it, strongly attracted by what I perceived to be its almost mathematical structure based on roots.

After reading two books on the literary analysis of the Hebrew Bible — *The Art of Biblical Narrative* by Robert Alter and *Slayers of Moses: The Emergence of Rabbinic Interpretation in Modern Literary Theory* by Susan A. Handelman — I realized that I was able to apply to its narratives and poetry the literary skills that had lain dormant for years. The Hebrew Bible was not the dead, legal treatise I had thought it was in my youth. After living in Israel, I came to realize that the Hebrew Bible was a vibrant literature of the spirit, sacred not because God had written it — a concept I do not understand — but because the Hebrew language in which it was written allowed it to create an open-ended, intricately interwoven, and gloriously ambiguous text pregnant with infinite possibilities. As I would later learn, and as we will see in chapters 4–6, in many places the Hebrew Bible speaks a Buddhist language that goes beyond words and concepts, a textual analog of the Buddhist way of living. By being mindful of its artful use of words, literary devices, the interplay of themes, narrative point of view, imagery, and the like, I found myself able to analyze the Hebrew Bible as literature.

With the support of my rabbi, Sheila Weinberg, I began teaching the Hebrew Bible at our synagogue in Amherst. At about the same time I became active in Jewish affairs at the University of Massachusetts. These efforts and my knowledge of the Bible led to a position as an adjunct professor in the Department of

Judaic and Near Eastern Studies. There I have taught courses on the Hebrew Bible, the Book of Job, and the writings of Franz Kafka. I also published articles on the Hebrew Bible, literature, and the Holocaust, and for three years I taught an adult education course on Jewish texts.

The Hebrew Bible and Buddhist teachings are two fountains of wisdom that did more than nourish me. They sustained me during the multiple crises that spanned two decades. The headache attack of 1980, which I treated using relaxation techniques based on Buddhist meditation, foreshadowed the much more acute headache attack of 2000 that is a focus of this book. In turn, the crisis caused by the second attack mirrored, distorted, reconfigured, and reinterpreted the crisis caused by the math book in 1985, which exposed as illusions many of my deeply held beliefs about achievement, creativity, and the mind.

As I look back on the experience of the math book, it is clear that there was no way out. My ego was too entangled in this project that teased me with a perfectibility I was unable to consummate. I dug and dug to discover that ultimate truth, ultimate perfection are unattainable. This was a major insight encompassing much more than just mathematics. During the months preceding the publication of the book, I gazed deeply into the guts of a purgatory described by Pascal in his *Pensées*:

> We are floating in a medium of vast extent, always drifting uncertainly, blown to and fro; whenever we think we have a fixed point to which we can cling and make fast, it shifts and leaves us behind; if we follow it, it eludes our grasp, slips away, and flees eternally before us. Nothing stands still for

us. This is our natural state and yet the state most contrary to our inclinations. We burn with desire to find a firm footing, an ultimate, lasting base on which to build a tower rising up to infinity, but our whole foundation cracks and the earth opens up into the depth of the abyss.

My experience with the math book could have been an opening for me. I could have turned to religion, as Pascal did. I could have gone with the flow, recognizing the mystery, the unknowability, the impossibility of finding a fixed point to which I could cling and make fast, and living with this wisdom. But it took years before the Buddha could help me translate Pascal into the language of my life.

In 1985 I was tottering on the edge of the abyss that the book had gashed open deep inside me, and I almost fell in. Despite the extent of my suffering, this experience was not enough of an impetus to cause me to change. Before I could assimilate Pascal's wisdom, during the 1980s I would have to live in Jerusalem and discover my Israeli family and relearn Hebrew and start to write the novel. During the 1990s I would have to be breathed by God at a Jewish-Buddhist meditation retreat and would have to send both of my children off to college and write my second math book and teach the Hebrew Bible and publish several essays. And in the fateful year 2000, as I was completing a research paper on statistical mechanical models of turbulence, the turbulence roiling just beneath the surface of my life for decades would finally have to erupt in the headache earthquake. One year later I would have to deal with my father's death, and the year after that, I would have to meet Jean Colucci, who would teach me the heart of meditation: separating myself from the pain is dualistic thinking, which in turn causes great suffering. Accepting the pain as my own was a key step in the process of observing the impermanence of self, which in turn led to my healing and to my letting go of the past.

Finally, mercifully, the past is over. In whatever ways I may have harmed myself, I offer myself forgiveness. In whatever ways I may have harmed others, I ask them for forgiveness. In whatever ways others may have harmed me, I offer them forgiveness.

2
Our Wounds Will Heal Us

> We are to think of the Buddha as a physician who cures not strictly physical ailments, but broadly psychological ones, who shows "wounded" human beings the way to the highest form of happiness.
> — Christopher W. Gowans, *Philosophy of the Buddha*

WHEN THE HEADACHES ERUPTED in 2000, I was in a deep sleep. Three and a half years later, I was visited by two Buddhist insights that would lead to my healing and my waking up. The truth is in my pain. The truth is in my face. It is the truth of the end of suffering and of mindfulness as a path that leads to the end of suffering.

This truth is so simple, yet so deep. It did not come from my rational, planning, hyperactive mind, on which I had relied all of my life. As Lama Tashi Namgyal explains in the introduction to *Medicine Buddha Teachings*, these insights were a manifestation of "the innate healing powers inherent in the basic nature of all sentient beings," uncovered and accessed through meditation:

> According to the teachings of the Buddha Shakyamuni, recorded in the *Sutra on Entering*

the Womb, there are four classes of illness. . . . The third class of illness includes those for which medicines are of no use, illnesses from which one cannot recover simply through the use of medicines or other medical procedures. These illnesses, however, can be cured — and one can thereby recover one's health — through the practice of appropriate spiritual techniques taught in the buddhadharma. . . . Through such practices, the innate healing powers inherent in the basic nature of all sentient beings can be uncovered and accessed.

The narrative in this chapter will ferry us across the void separating the headaches from the healing. As I was crossing that void alone on my rickety raft of meditation, it seemed to be infinitely wide. But in reality, the opposite shore was just a breath away. This is my story, embedded in the details of my life yet addressing universal themes: the desperation of blinding pain; serious side effects from the pills prescribed by many doctors; dealing with the pain by distraction, avoidance, and fear; being overwhelmed with self-pity; slowly returning to meditation; seeking help from a therapist; attending a meditation retreat at which the truth of the pain was revealed; gratitude and deepening meditation practice. If you have suffered, whether from physical pain, emotional pain, or the dissatisfaction and sense of lack that is pervasive in our lives, then I expect that you will recognize aspects of these themes in your own experience.

The headaches erupted on a dark night in February 2000. A wild winter wind howling, I awakened, afraid to awaken. Lightning. Thunder. Whirlwind. Flame. A storm of Biblical enormity short-circuiting the fuses in my face. An earthquake savaging my forehead, splitting open my skull with jack-hammering pain. All the changes and losses and rejections of the past months, the past years, the past lifetimes focusing their raw fury on the nerves between my eyes, the nerves igniting and burning with a chronic, neuralgic hellfire. Eyeglasses became impossible to wear. The pressure of even the most lightweight pair caused insufferable pain to radiate through my forehead and nose. Dear God, please help me. My face is on fire. My life is my work, but I can't even read.

Desperate, I went from doctor to doctor. One neurologist misdiagnosed me and prescribed a heavy dose of a dangerous drug. An otolaryngologist advised injecting Botox or, if that didn't work, severing a major facial nerve. A psychiatrist, week after week, told me that I was seething with anger. Another neurologist, who I will call Dr. B., applied a trans-nasal Lidocaine nerve block of my sphenopalatine ganglion, which made the pain much worse, and in response to that, prescribed heavy doses of multiple medications. Dr. B., as my wife Alison saw but I didn't, was a brusque and pompous mechanic for whom my body was a pill receptacle and for whom I was a nuisance. In the worst tradition of Western medicine, he loaded me with drugs that in masking some of the pain, sucked up all my intellectual and emotional energy.

I suffered from the pain and even more from my outrage over the pain. The truth was in my face, but I didn't see it. Duped by the medical profession and deceived by my own blindness, I cried out, "Where should I turn?" No one answered. I shouted, "How can I get relief?" Nothing worked. "What if the pain gets much worse?" I shrieked. The pain mocked me by throbbing even more.

Tension and stress exacerbated the pain. Being a mathematician who worshipped at the altar of reason, I logically tried to protect myself from all tension and stress. But despite my

Herculean efforts, I realized that I couldn't control the world. A diary entry from that period shows how deep my suffering was:

> Went to bed last night with a bad headache. Took two aspirins before retiring. Headache only got worse. Took a Fiorinal and moved to the guest bedroom. An hour later, pain still bad. Watched *Groundhog Day* for the nth time and took another Fiorinal. Whatever works to get my mind off this curse. Fell asleep, but slept fitfully. Up at 7 AM, raging pain in my forehead and nose. Waited until Alison left. Afraid she might say something that will set me off.

Pills, distraction, avoidance, fear. Unskillful tools for dealing with the pain, whose monkey mind was much more clever than my own. Whenever I tried to push it away, it punished me by plunging me into its raging inferno.

The summer of 2000 was my summer of crisis. I — graduate of Harvard in mathematics and German literature; Professor of Mathematics; Adjunct Professor of Judaic Studies; mathematician with a theorem named after me; self-taught Bible exegete and teacher; author of high-level math books, articles on literature, and a novel I couldn't publish — I became the dried-out shell of the passionate person I had been since the days of my youth.

I was in the grip of an uncontrollable fear. What if this pain lasts forever? Miraculously, or perhaps because I was in such deep need, memories of a weekend of deep connection percolated into my consciousness. It was the weekend spent six years earlier in 1994 at a Jewish-Buddhist meditation retreat in Barre, Massachusetts.

Energized by my fear during the summer of 2000, I fabricated a refuge out of those memories. Inside that refuge I carefully nurtured the insights that in 1994 had blossomed within me and that I had carefully recorded. The insight that the myriad tasks life presents me need not be sources of anxiety, but can be opportunities to cultivate mindfulness. The insight that in meditation the mind returns to its natural relaxed state, allowing one to see things as they really are. The insight that, like the breath, everything passes. The insight, preposterous from the perspective of dualistic thinking yet experientially obvious, that the universe is breathing through me without my control or intervention. That I am being breathed. That I am being lived. And most liberating of all: the insight that the struggle can be over and I can let go because God, the source of all being, is everywhere.

In desperation during the summer of 2000, I read through those insights, groping for even a filament of wisdom that might keep me from drowning. But I failed. As the Buddha said in the *Dhammapada* (translation by Eknath Easwaran), "Our life is shaped by our mind; we become what we think. Suffering follows an evil thought as the wheels of a cart follow the oxen that draw it." As I quickly realized, my hope of rekindling the spirit of the Jewish-Buddhist retreat in Barre and keeping it alive were doomed. The insights that had blossomed during my three days there could not purify my mind of the poisons with which my 17,000 days of conditioning had polluted it.

During the summer of 2000 I was haunted by questions. O pure light of Barre, where did you go? Did you follow our son Michael when he went off to Yale three years ago or our daughter Melissa when she fell in love and graduated from Yale and entered medical school, my body aging, Alison's body aging, my mother becoming ill, my father's body nourishing the colon cancer that would take his life within the next year?

Rejections were everywhere. Despite my many contributions to mathematics, invitations to speak at conferences slowed to a trickle. Even worse, in early 2000 my National Science Foundation proposal was not funded for only the second time in thirty years, and a few weeks later I found out, despite all expectations to the contrary, that I was not awarded a prestigious faculty fellowship at my university, and my 479-page math book co-written with Paul Dupuis and published in 1997 — a project on which we had slaved for years — brought us no recognition, and I couldn't publish my novel despite years of trying. The ego that needed to be protected and stroked was being mocked and mauled by a world that didn't care.

There were also many successes and great fulfillment. However, as the new year 2000 dawned, I was blind to the blessings of my life. My beautiful daughter Melissa would be married in May to a terrific guy, who was also Jewish. Although I did not see it at the time, I was not ready to let her go. And I suffered.

When the headaches started, I cursed and raged against the pain, but my cursing and raging made it much worse, solidifying the pain into the only conceptual lens for interpreting my moment-to-moment experience. Thus conditioned, my mind made the inevitable choice, which in turn locked it into a never-ending cycle of aversion and attachment. What increases my pain is bad and is to be avoided. What decreases my pain is good and is to be clung to.

I tried to take pleasure in the achievements I had spent a lifetime garnering. But they were vanity and ego. Like the drugs I was taking, they were incapable of extinguishing the fire that smoldered in the middle of my face. What did I do to deserve this torture? Who am I? Where am I? Who was shouting from the great and mighty wind raging around me, splitting mountains and shattering rocks? How accurately the words of the First Book of Kings described my struggle (translation by Rabbi Lawrence Kushner in his essay "Breathing"):

> And lo, the LORD passed by. There was a great and mighty wind, splitting mountains and shattering rocks by the power of the LORD; but the LORD was not in the wind. After the wind, an earthquake; but the LORD was not in the earthquake. After the earthquake, fire; but the LORD was not in the fire. And after the fire, the soft barely audible sound of almost breathing. (I Kings 19:11–12)

A stranger to my wife and to myself, tyrannized by my pain, yet struggling to keep a normal exterior so that no one else could gauge my suffering, in July 2000 I consulted with another neurologist, who assured me that the MRI of my brain was normal — no tumor, no cancer. After informing me that he had no idea how the pain started and why it was still hurting and when, if ever, it would go away, Dr. Venna urged me to try to taper Dr. B.'s pharmacopoeia of personality-altering drugs. My goal was not to be pain-free by overmedicating myself, but to find a manageable level of pain with a minimum of drugs.

Inspired by the interaction with my new neurologist, I heard the soft barely audible sound of almost breathing across the chasm and through the chaos of the six Biblical years of suffering since the 1994 retreat in Barre. Dr. Nagagopal Venna had grown up in the land of the Buddha. The Buddha. Meditation. In meditation the mind returns to its natural relaxed state. Like the breath everything passes. The universe is breathing through me without my control or intervention. The struggle can be over and I can let go because God, the source of all being, is everywhere. And through the chaos, Alison was always present. But I had become blind to her wisdom and her love.

The radiance of the insights that had blossomed at Barre and somehow resurfaced through the noise and the pain could not penetrate the thick shell encasing my heart, which was locked in a struggle against the drugs, each reduction bringing more pain, and against the pain, torturously and exquisitely aggravated by stress, stress lurking in every interaction, particularly those with Alison, to whose innocent comments about my appearance or actions I often strongly reacted, my reactivity triggering stress that registered as more pain that I blamed on her because I was not yet aware of the intimate karmic connection between the reactivity and the stress into which only great effort over the next few years would give me insight, my blame, in turn, triggering her to react, resulting in yet more stress and more pain and more blame. The maelstrom of *dukkha* kept sucking me in as it spun faster and faster.

In December 2000, the Amitriptyline and the Doxycycline and the Nortriptyline and the Neurontin and the Klonapin and the Clonazepam having been successfully weaned from my system, the pain alarmingly flared up, rekindling the fire in the middle of my face that congealed into a sharp, pinching nose-pain that glowed white hot. Why couldn't anybody see it? This was the mark of Cain, branded into my face as a punishment for eradicating my old self. "A restless wanderer shall you be," thundered God, pounding the rusty nail into the bone between my eyes, clamping the razor-edged plier-jaws just below my nose-bridge, the pressure throbbing with each breath.

Could meditation help? In desperation I tried, but the pain polluted my noble efforts. A typical scene. I find a comfortable chair and shut my eyes and follow my breath, noting that the pain isn't bad today, just a wave of sensation rolling between my eyes. Breath in. Breath out. Breath in, getting caught in the wave, which becomes angry and surges down the damaged nerve into my nasal passage — I can't stop it although I know what is about to happen — and transmogrifies there into the sharp, pinching clamped-plier-throbbing-pressure of nose pain that is so sharp that following my breath mindfully becomes as impossible as excising my nose from my face, which I'd really like to do because it hurts so fucking bad.

The meditation tape I was listening to lied. It said that meditation is the solution, but for me it was the problem. Regardless of the pain's intensity when I sat down, the act of meditation made it only worse. The pain knew my agenda — that I was meditating to get rid of it — and the pain always outfoxed me. The tape said that meditation has no agenda, that in returning the mind to its natural relaxed state, one can see things as they really are. The landscape of my mind was painted with pain. Why would I want to see that?

Months passed, and the screws tightened. My father died. My mother, brother, and I buried him, and I mourned him because I loved him, and I cried because we had never been close. My parents' house was sold, and my brother and I helped Mom move, and her health was not good. Against that onslaught the meditation was a waste of time. By increasing the one drug I was still taking, I was able to reduce the pain to a manageable level, but whatever its level, the pain pissed me off. Enough already.

Whatever I did to deserve it, my debt had been paid, my life still a turmoil, frequent attacks of facial pain compounded by events spinning out of control.

How relentlessly the wheel kept turning. Our new furnace filling the basement with a stinking, sulfurous stench that no repairman could fix; trouble with a course I was teaching; no breakthroughs in my research and two new research proposals to write; mistakenly erasing all my computer files in an act of cyber-suicide and spending half a day frantically restoring them instead of being with Melissa, who was visiting us at the time; disagreeing with Alison during the two-hour ride home from Boston over how best to care for my mother and how I could have dealt better with my father and how Alison wished that I'd stop talking about my pain so much because talking about it made it worse.

That disagreement rekindled the memories of my father's death more than a year earlier. I sat next to his bed in the nursing home not knowing what to say. Who was this man who had passed on to me his love of books but couldn't show his love for me, rejecting me for years and now dying this painful death by colon cancer that had metastasized to the liver? I took his hand and rubbed it.

"Richard, you never held my hand before."

It was the most emotional statement I ever heard him say. Through my tears I whispered, "Dad, I love you," while kissing his hot brow. He died on the first night of Passover 2001. But his death did not liberate me from the Egypt of our broken relationship. That would have to wait for more than seven years until I visited his grave and forgave him and through him, myself.

But I couldn't forgive my father in April 2000. Just before Melissa's wedding he made an accusation on the phone about our relationship that cut me like a knife. When Alison and I got home after that ride from Boston, his voice kept screaming, forcing me to justify my existence, forcing me to shout back, "Why did you attack me?", and my face throbbed with pain that would probably last forever. Alison and I went to bed, I couldn't sleep, I got up, his voice was getting louder, I moved to another bed. His voice kept screaming and I screamed back because I couldn't listen to him and my forehead was pounding, pounding, pounding, about to burst. Quiet the whole ride home as I parried his attacks like a karate master, my ego was now ablaze, lashing me to a whipping post and pistol-whipping me, eyes bulging and nostrils flared. My father was dead. I wanted my father to love me. At a time when I needed him so much, he attacked me. My ego incinerated me and revived me only to fling me against the stone wall of my anger and picked me up bleeding and retching and flung me again and again. No sleep at all.

 On September 1, 2002, no closer to figuring out the pain than when it had erupted two and a half years earlier, I again sought help. Like Dr. Venna, whom I had found almost by chance, I found Jean Colucci, a clinician who based her therapy on Buddhist principles and agreed to work with me.

 "Is there a way out of this confusion?" I asked Jean.

 "Yes," she replied. "Mindfulness."

 I was skeptical, but nothing else was working.

 A few weeks after the therapy had started, I tried again to meditate. With Jean's encouragement I was able to do it except when there was too much pain. Then it happened. One evening at dinner Alison brought up the visit to my mother the day before. I hadn't talked much there, and as I realized even before Alison spoke, I could have been more sympathetic to how my mother was feeling. It was the kind of conversation that even a few months earlier I would not have let go of, precipitating a fight that might have lasted for days. But this time, awake and aware, I apologized without trying to protect myself or explain myself. My conversation with Alison was just words. The memory of the visit to my mother was just a breath that would fade if I let it go. The seeds that had been planted in Barre in 1994 bore their first fruit. And the fruit became an orchard as one month, two months went by without even a disagreement between my wife and me. Our love began to flourish again, as it had in our youth.

Insight led to insight. At the 1994 retreat someone had recommended that I attend the mindfulness-based stress-reduction course developed by Jon Kabat-Zinn at the University of Massachusetts Medical School in Worcester, about an hour from my house. The seed planted by this person flowered during my sabbatical in the spring of 2003, which I spent in a manner faithful to the root meaning of the word. Like God on the seventh day, I rested from my labors during that spring. Among other gifts, the course in Worcester gave me the understanding and discipline that motivated me to undertake a daily meditation practice.

This led to the next breakthrough, which would not have happened without Alison's understanding and support. After months of slowly tapering my last medication, a pill that was effective against the pain but was potentially harmful to my liver, in May 2003 I stopped taking the medication completely. I celebrated by flushing down the toilet the hundreds of remaining pills that had accumulated. Thank you, Dr. Venna and Jean and the stress-reduction course in Worcester, for the blessings of meditation and therapy, and thank you, my darling wife, for your quiet wisdom and constant love, to which I was slowly awakening.

Mindfulness spread its deep roots. One morning in the spring after meditating, I realized that for the first time since the 1994 retreat I was experiencing prolonged periods of relaxation and peace even while being thoroughly immersed in life's tasks. Meditation was both the sun and the fertile soil, allowing the insights that had blossomed in Barre and then disappeared, to bloom again after nearly a decade of dead ends and silent growth, mindlessness and mindfulness, suffering and healing.

Appropriately, Barre was again the locus for my next life-enhancing insight. In August 2003, while attending an eight-day retreat at the Insight Meditation Society, the sharp, pinching clamped-plier-throbbing-pressure of nose pain ambushed me at 3:30 AM on the second morning. Shit, I shouted as I pounded the wall of my room, feeling vulnerable and very scared, my soul exposed to the pain's merciless throbbing from which, especially at Barre, there was no escape. I came here for enlightenment and still have to deal with this fucking pain. What if it never goes away?

I was on the verge of abandoning the retreat and coming home, but I forced myself to go to the first sitting, where I followed the advice of one of the leaders of the retreat. Rather than focus on my pain, I focused on the pressure of my feet on the ground. The pain suddenly decreased, at times almost disappearing. At the level of bare awareness stripped of all drama and self-pity, I perceived that the pressure in my nose equaled the pressure of gravity on my feet. I don't wish for gravity to disappear, so why make a similar demand of the pain?

The next morning, the pain ebbing and flowing across the lower forehead into the left nostril and back again, I begged it to spare me. O God, please let it go away. I have suffered enough. During the sitting just before lunch, without any conscious effort on my part, I was shocked to discover the insights of the previous day deepening to gratitude — no, love — for the headaches. A voice in my head was speaking to the pain. "You have taught me so much about myself and my place in the interconnected web of life. You have brought me to meditation and to therapy, which in turn have opened me up to the spiritual roots of my suffering. You are my third eye, the wisdom source in the center of my face. My pain, my honored teacher, please forgive me. I have spent three and a half years pushing you away, cursing you, creating duality, exacerbating the discomfort with aversion. Pain, I love you," I said silently in the meditation hall. "What else will you teach me today? My goal is to love you and then to let you go."

Out of the blue, two phrases manifested themselves in my mind. The truth is in my pain. The truth is in my face. As soon as I grasped for the handles to unlock the meaning of these phrases, I became aware of this grasping and let it go. I knew that the meaning would unfold for me when I was ready.

During lunch the phrase "love it and let it go" kept running through my head. Let go of the pain. Let go of Melissa. Let go of myself. Let go of my grasping, holding, hoarding, selfish self. I wanted to cry. Unable to eat, I returned to my room, lay down in bed, and sobbed. For three and a half years, the truth had been in my face, in both senses of the phrase. On Tuesday, August 5, 2003, I finally saw it.

During the early sitting on Wednesday morning, for the first time in years I meditated with my head almost totally pain-free.

As I write this, more than a decade has passed since the 1994 retreat. The pain is still here, but the pain is not the issue because happiness does not depend upon external conditions and the content of experience. Rather, happiness depends on how I respond to experience. It depends upon my level of mindfulness, upon my level of accepting that the truth is in my pain. The multifold meanings of this insight continue to unfold for me. I, who have so wanted to control life, cannot control life. I cannot control the pain, which has a mind of its own.

As I finally learned, the Buddha's Second Noble Truth explained my suffering, which arose because I craved to get rid of the pain. Not understanding that pain is a concept, I congealed the pain into a solid, substantial reality and then suffered from that solidification. In the introduction to *Medicine Buddha Teachings,* Lama Tashi Namgyal describes this process:

> All phenomena are ephemeral, constantly changing in the same way as the appearances within a kaleidoscope constantly change. None of these illusory appearances — including the appearances of sickness and disease, which are also mere empty appearances — has the power to cause us suffering unless we mistakenly apprehend them as real and substantial. When we misapprehend these appearances, when we take them to be real, we fixate on them, and thereby cause them to solidify in our experience. This gives them the appearance of solid, substantial reality, and then in our lives these illness do, in fact, become for us very real and solid, and we suffer from them.

When the pain began in February 2000, I identified with it. I cursed it. Fearful and despairing, I tried to push it away. Two and a half millennia ago the Buddha described exactly how I acted and how I felt in his teaching about the arrow (translation by Thanissaro Bhikkhu):

> When touched with a feeling of pain, the uninstructed run-of-the-mill person sorrows, grieves, and laments, beats his breast, becomes distraught. So he feels two pains, physical and mental. Just as if they were to shoot a man with an arrow and, right afterward, were to shoot him with another one, so that he would feel the pains of two arrows.

I came to understand that pain and suffering are not synonymous. My meditation practice has taught me the difference. As Stephen Cope explains in his book, *The Wisdom of Yoga*, pain cannot be avoided, but suffering, *dukkha*, can:

> We each have pain. It comes with the territory of being a human being. And pain that is fully experienced is, of course, painful. But suffering — *duhkka* [sic] — is something different. *Duhkha* is *resistance* to that pain. *Duhkha* is the reactivity to that pain. *Duhkha* is what Chögyam Trungpa Rinpoche called "the pain of pain." As the Buddhist teacher Sylvia Boorstein says, "Pain is inevitable. Suffering is optional."

These insights are corollaries of the first three Noble Truths: there is suffering; suffering arises from aversion; suffering can end. Here is a mathematical formulation, elegant and succinct, of these Noble Corollaries in the calculus of suffering, which took me years to penetrate (adapted from "Psychophysiological Disorders: Embracing Pain" by Ronald D. Siegel):

suffering ≠ pain;
suffering = pain × resistance;
if resistance = 0, then suffering = 0.

My headaches responded to meditation as taught by the Buddha, not to medication as dispensed by Dr. B. As I was writing this chapter, I received an invitation to attend a conference on headaches and chronic facial pain. Numerous sessions on a variety of topics were planned: dental vs. neuropathic facial pain, side effects of medication, the value of complementary and alternative medicine, microvascular decompression, radiosurgery, motor cortex stimulation. Meditation is not mentioned.

As meditation has taught me to transform the pain from a concept into an energy flow, so I also try to live my life. By being a verb and not a noun, a jazz riff and not a symphony. By being open to nuance and surprise and change. By not investing words and experiences with fixed meanings, but by recognizing that they are empty. This Buddhist concept conveys not a meaningless void, but a dynamic, interconnected web of significance devoid of any defining essence and therefore, like the words of the Hebrew Bible, pregnant with possibility. I can't force a coherent narrative on my pain, so why do it with my life? I want to let my life flourish in its ambiguity and its multiple interpretability and its occasional incoherence. I want to play with my life as I play with the text of the holy Hebrew Bible and, in playing with it, become God's partner.

As my Buddhist practice deepens to touch more and more facets of my being, I embrace the suffering Richard S. Ellis of November 1994, who for three days stepped outside his busy, unfocused life to be breathed by God at the Barre Center for Buddhist Studies. Recalling that experience, I repeat the words of our forefather Jacob, grateful for understanding how his words describe my evolution. Upon awakening from his dream in which he saw messengers of God going up and down a ladder, Jacob exclaimed, "Indeed the LORD is in this place, and I did not know" (Gen. 28:16).*

In this place. This place is my face. The truth is in my face. In this place, in my face, my pain has opened me up to hear God, the same God who was in the earthquake of February 2000 that savaged my forehead and was in the hellfire with which my face burned after the lightning storm had short-circuited the nerves between my eyes. Finally I can hear God whispering to me what God spoke to the Prophet Jeremiah: "Wake up. I will heal you with your wounds" (Jer. 30:17).

As Buddhist meditation teaches us, our wounds are not a noun. They are a verb. Breathe in. Breathe out. The entire world in our in-breath. The pain, our honored teacher, can become our lens for understanding this and all the Buddhist teachings. The truth is in our pain. The truth is in our face. It's so simple, yet so deep. A lightning bolt of insight revealed the truth to me while meditating at the Insight Meditation Society on August 5, 2003. In the next chapter I tell the story of how this insight liberated me from the prison of my suffering on that summer day when the sky was huge and blue and one could gaze into the deepest expanse of the universe if one just opened one's eyes.

Whether you suffer from chronic pain or from the dissatisfaction and sense of lack that is symptomatic of the human condition, my hope is that reading about my *dukkha* will help you become more deeply aware of yours. May the calm light of awareness lead to insight, transformation, and peace.

---

* Unless otherwise indicated, all translations from the Five Books of Moses are taken from Robert Alter's *The Five Books of Moses: A Translation with Commentary*.

3
Waking Up to the Truth

> Do not explore the future. Rather, whatever
> happens to you accept with perfect trust.
> — Rashi, commentary on Deut. 18:13

THROUGH NO EFFORT OF MY OWN, a flash of insight woke me up on August 5, 2003. While meditating that morning at the Insight Meditation Society in Barre, Massachusetts, I intuitively understood that the truth about the pain is in my face. After years of hating the pain, that morning I started to love it, allowing the pain eventually to become my best teacher. However, I had to prepare the way. Although the flash of insight came through no effort of my own, it would not have happened if I had not been practicing meditation regularly during the previous months.

This chapter, intimate and introspective, is the heart of the book because it addresses one of the central experiences of Buddhist practice: how we can end suffering by quieting the mind and giving truth the space to speak. What spoke to me that morning, and what can speak to you if you are open and ready, was an innate voice of wisdom, our Buddha nature, normally obscured by noise and distraction. Though embedded in the details of my life, my experience can be your experience.

This was not my first awakening in Barre. The first time was in November 1994 when, at the Barre Center for Buddhist Studies, I realized that I am being breathed and being lived by the universe, by God, by the source of all breath. Despite the force of that insight, I fell asleep again for almost nine years as soon as I returned home.

The circumstances of the two awakenings were completely different. In 1994 I plunged from the maelstrom of a hyper-stressed, unaware life into the still waters of a Jewish-Buddhist retreat and back again into the maelstrom as soon as the retreat had ended. My mind was so conditioned by the frantic pace that my awakening quickly dissipated into the shadow of a memory of connectedness and openness having no resonance, afterlife, or force. As I was drowning, I tried to record the shadow of that memory a few days after the retreat had ended. But the words detached themselves from my experiences as soon as they hit the page.

In contrast, the eight-day retreat of August 2003 crowned a sabbatical semester that I honored in the root meaning of the word. Like God on the Sabbath, I rested during that semester of introspection, meditation, and therapy. During the retreat, I suffered from some of the worst pain since the headaches had erupted. Despite the headaches, or perhaps because of them, on August 5 I awakened from my nine-year slumber when I realized, with a joy of insight unmediated by any conceptual lens, the truth about my pain, a truth that continues to resonate until today.

The 1994 Jewish-Buddhist Contemplative Dialogue was held at the Barre Center for Buddhist Studies during three days in November. It was the third annual retreat celebrating Jewish renewal. The retreat was led by Rabbi Sheila Weinberg, who at the time was the rabbi of the Jewish Community of Amherst, where I am a member, and by Sylvia Boorstein, who introduced herself as a meditation teacher, a wife, a mother, and a grandmother. I felt close to Sheila, having studied Jewish texts with her and having discussed personal matters on numerous occasions. Two years earlier she had officiated at my son's bar mitzvah, and six years later she would officiate at my daughter's wedding.

When I sat down to dinner on Thursday, three days ahead of me without an agenda, I took a deep breath and audibly sighed. I felt so tired. This seemed to be the first time since the summer that I had stopped working. What did I do last summer for fun? It was a faded memory. Too sensitive to criticism. Overburdened with everything I had to do. Annoyed that I had to put my work on hold so that I could attend this retreat. So much ego to protect and to stroke. My second math book, on which Paul Dupuis and I had been working for years, caused me to push myself almost to the limit of my ego-driven energy in order to prove my worth after a lifetime of continually proving it, as if another book or another achievement could have any positive effect on the state of my soul. My ego was a pit that could never be filled.

The Thursday night program was led by Sylvia in the new meditation building. Leaving my sandals in the shoe room and entering the meditation hall inside, I gasped in wonder at its beauty. The floor was made of polished, aromatic wood, and the high, vaulted ceiling was supported by crisscrossing beams of the same color wood as the floor. The wisdom flowed from Sylvia, not in a glib way, but sincerely and quietly and thus powerfully. But I was not quiet inside, and her words quickly vanished. We ended the evening with meditation practice. I had trouble sitting still for more than a few minutes.

In bed by 10 PM that first night, I followed Sylvia's instructions not to read and not to write but to remain inward. My God, what about my work? When would I get it all done? I smiled to myself. Since dinner, this was the first time I had thought about it.

All of Friday was devoted to silence. The plan was that as Sabbath approached — or rather, Shabbos, as everyone called it, using the softer Yiddish word — we would enter into speech and song. Friday morning was devoted to sitting. As time went on, I was able to sit longer and longer. But I was never really comfortable, and I could not decide whether to sit on a chair or on the floor or, while sitting on the floor, whether to use one cushion or two or whether to interfold my legs in the lotus position as many participants were doing. Whenever I tried it, my legs soon ached. It was painfully apparent that I was the least skilled meditator there.

As I sat in the meditation hall, I glanced at the circular window at the far end. The hall was so quiet that the flies buzzing against the glass could be heard. The flies have no concept of glass and therefore no idea what keeps them trapped inside. We too are flies butting our heads against the windowpanes of our egos, which keep us trapped inside. What fools we are, locked in our conceptual prisons. Rather than seek to liberate ourselves, we use our energy to protect our egos, making the windowpanes of our prisons only thicker.

Sylvia instructed us on how to follow the breath, encouraging us to keep our senses open. "In meditation we experience the natural relaxed state of the mind. We experience freedom a breath at a time. And if we can experience freedom moment to moment, then we have it for eternity because moments are all we have." It was soothing and wise. Each of the sittings during the retreat ended when Sylvia sounded the brass gong at her feet. When I was able to quiet my mind, I could hear the sound of the gong reverberate for many seconds.

On Friday morning I had an insight. It was windy outside as a storm was gathering force. I was listening to the wind and following my breath, and I felt the world breathing through me. My breathing was involuntary as the energy of the universe passed through my lungs without my control or intervention. I am being breathed. I am being lived. I am being breathed by the universe, by God, by the source of all breath, and therefore I can let go. Freedom is a breath away. Where were my concerns that raged the evening before? A bonfire from which I was removing the fuel, they were slowly disappearing.

At the end of the sitting I shared my insight about the breath with Sylvia, who validated it as fundamental. I looked at Sheila, who was standing nearby. She nodded her head and smiled. Sylvia and Sheila and me and all the other participants and Mu Soeng, the Buddhist monk who welcomed us as we entered the building this morning — God breathed us all into being:

> [T]hen the LORD God fashioned the human, humus from the soil, and blew into his nostrils the breath of life, and the human became a living creature. (Gen. 2:7)

During lunch I was overwhelmed with my insight about the breath and thought about it extensively, not tasting my food. Half an hour later I completely forgot what I had eaten. The afternoon was devoted to Metta, the Buddhist practice of lovingkindness. We were instructed to say to ourselves the following words: "I want to be safe. I want to be happy. I want to be healthy. I want to be at ease." After directing the kind thoughts to ourselves, we were to direct them to the person or persons about whom we have the most expansive and the most open feelings. I thought of my wife and my children back home in Amherst, an hour and a world away.

On Friday night Shabbos began at the Buddhist Center with lighting candles. Sheila was standing next to me and hugged me as I lit mine. As the light was enlightening my soul, the power of the moment was enhanced by my memory of the hour walk I had just completed amidst the muted colors of mid-November. We sang Shabbos songs. The words did not make as strong an impression as the feeling of real joy among us seekers.

Sheila shared with us a question asked by one of the participants. What in Jewish practice corresponds to the Buddhist practice of Metta? She turned to Peter, whose full grey beard accentuated the light streaming from his gentle eyes. Peter seemed able to sit quietly for hours, meditating while Sheila and Sylvia spoke, even while the rest of us were just lolling around. Sheila asked Peter to tell the group what he had told her; namely, that the priestly benediction — *Yevorechecha Adonay ve-yishmerecha* — was the Jewish Metta. He then gave a sensitive, Buddhist-inspired translation:

> May God protect you. May you be safe.
> May God enlighten you. May you be enlightened.
> May you see God's face in every face you see and
> thus find peace.

While Peter was speaking, a woman about my age lay down, fell asleep, and began to snore. People tried to awaken her, and everyone around her became extremely perturbed. I could not help but laugh to myself. We came to Barre for enlightenment but had to deal with this snoring person. Aside from farting out loud in the meditation hall, snoring was the worst sin. The next morning the woman would wake up. She would joyfully dance with the Torah scroll, wearing a smile from ear to ear.

Rather than eat breakfast on Saturday at the Buddhist Center, I ate at the guest house where I was staying. I was joined by a woman named Sarah and two other women. Sarah commented on the Holocaust, the first of many references during the retreat to that never-to-be-healed wound in the collective Jewish soul. Because of the Holocaust, she said, the Jewish people were still going through post-traumatic shock. Hitler had murdered most of our spiritual leaders, who took their treasures with them to the grave.

"Not everything was lost," one of the other women said. Although I had just been introduced to her, I was embarrassed to have forgotten her name already. "I came to this retreat," she continued, "to revive in my soul the sparks of holiness that my grandmother of blessed memory has transmitted to me from beyond her grave. She lived in Vilna, Lithuania, where the Nazis slaughtered her and her family."

A long silence followed while I, and presumably the others around the table, absorbed the potency of this revelation.

Sarah told a story that she had heard from an Orthodox man concerning why women should not be allowed to hold the Torah scroll. " 'The Torah,' he explained, 'is such a female symbol. We take it from the ark, we caress it, undress it, kiss it, we open it up, enter it, and we gain wisdom.' " All eyes were on Sarah. " 'A woman dancing with the Torah scroll is thus obviously a lesbian, and that is an abomination.' " Sarah burst into laughter — and we all joined in — over the blasphemy, from the mouth of an Orthodox man, of interacting sexually with the holy Torah. It was a brilliant insight, which recalled a teaching from Jewish mysticism: proper sexual relations between a man and a woman induce proper sexual relations between the male and female aspects of God.

I arrived at the Buddhist Center in time for the Shabbos service, which was to be the most powerful and joyous and connecting service I had ever participated in. The silence of the previous day now flowered into song. Such energy and happiness as we sang songs to celebrate being alive and being Jewish. After harmonizing with one of the standard Shabbos songs whose name didn't register because I was a wave on this ocean of joy, a woman from Amherst sang a lovely tune to the prayer "Where is the place of His honor?" The singing of the entire group was powerful and from the heart.

In the middle of the singing, it happened, the profound connection resonating with my insight of the day before. We chanted a prayer that I knew by heart, but it had never struck me with such intensity. "The soul of every living thing shall bless your name, ETERNAL ONE, Our God." The previous day's focus on meditation and the breath had sensitized me to the spirit of reverence breathing through this prayer. Then Sheila read aloud the long commentary by Rabbi Everett Gendler:

> *Nefesh, ruah, neshamah*: these three Hebrew terms are often translated as soul or spirit. They were originally terms for breath. This relation between soul and breathing is found in other sacred languages as well: *atman* in Sanskrit, *pneuma* in Greek, *anima* and *spiritus* in Latin are all terms for soul. All in origin refer to breath and breathing. Literally, then, this prayer asserts that the breath

of all living creatures proclaims God's blessing. In what sense might this be so?

I listened closely, holding my breath in anticipation of where the commentary was going. Sheila continued:

> Breath is the prerequisite of life and speech, of existence and communication, and it is a gift requiring no conscious attention except in cases of illness. If each inhalation required a direct order, each exhalation a conscious command, how should we find energy or attention for anything else? How should we sleep? In truth, we do not breathe; we are breathed. At this moment of my writing, at this moment of your reading, at succeeding moments of our praying, breath enters and leaves our lungs without our conscious intervention. Truly we are breathed.

Yes. Yes. I was soaring. This was identical to my insight of the day before. Listening to the wind. Following my breath. Feeling the world breathing through me, feeling the energy of the universe passing through my lungs without my control or intervention. I am being breathed. I am being lived. The struggle is over. Let the work go. Let the book go. Not just breathing, but all experience is empty of self. Reading the commentary and singing the melody that accompanied the prayer, I was soaring to a higher level of consciousness where I glimpsed the true nature of things.

Opening myself up to this prayer allowed yet more blessings to pour out upon me. Sensitized by the Buddhist teachings and the meditation practice, by the silence of the day before and the joy of this Shabbos service, I understood, intuitively and experientially, the inner meaning of the Shabbos prayers as they unfolded before me. Buddhism and Judaism are two converging paths to the unity of life and to the *neshamah* of the universe that breathes us.

During the Torah service, we passed the Torah scroll around. Everyone danced with it, and everyone was beaming. Upon the image of the Torah from breakfast as a woman whom we caress, undress, kiss, open, and enter to gain wisdom, another image was imposed. As each person in the group held the Torah scroll, it seemed to be a baby being cradled in each person's arm. Tears filled my eyes, and I started to cry.

After lunch, a woman named Eva shared with the group, in Hebrew-accented English, what arose for her during the Torah service. It concerned an uncle who had survived the Holocaust. In 1945 after the liberation, her uncle was visiting his father's grave somewhere in Europe. All of a sudden he realized that he wasn't wearing a head covering — a *kippah*, she called it, using the Hebrew word. He hadn't worn a *kippah* during the entire war because he had been a prisoner in Auschwitz. Out loud he exclaimed in Hebrew, "*Hitorarti*," meaning "I woke up." He reached into his pocket, knotted his handkerchief, and put it onto his head. Then he could visit his father's grave in peace. Eva ended by saying that, after an absence of more than twenty years, she had visited Israel during the previous year in order to learn more of the family history from her uncle, who told her this story. Soon thereafter her uncle died.

Another man at the service related that what came up for him was a vision of Jews being murdered during the Holocaust. "When I shut my eyes and listen," he said, "I hear the groans of our people in the ghettos and in the camps and in the gas chambers after the doors were locked shut and they realized what was happening. They die again and again, and each time I suffer." I was overwhelmed by the feeling that so many people in this room, including me, were similarly suffering from the Holocaust, even though most of us had been born after the war.

As this sharing was going on, I became the center of a circle of energy. Eva sat on my left, the Holocaust-sufferer on my right, a man from my synagogue behind me, Sylvia and Sheila a few feet away in front. The service continued, ending on a high level of connectedness and love. A young woman who had been turned onto Torah study by her father sang a beautiful piece about the beauty of the moment and how everything passes. The song forced me to see the truth: I didn't want the service to end, but it had to. Afterwards I spoke with Sheila and with Sylvia, who told me that I finally woke up, using the same words that Eva had used in her story.

All this energy and joy expanded my mind to an open, non-grasping, Shabbos consciousness. My ego disappeared. I was part of this group of seekers and singers, and my own self-centered concerns totally vanished.

Shabbos lunch was extremely spirited. While standing in line next to Eva as we waited for the food, I reflected aloud on the suffering caused by the Holocaust and mentioned what I have told only a few people. I have a strong feeling of having been reincarnated from the Holocaust. My soul was the soul of someone whom the Nazis had murdered.

Eva replied by describing an incident that had happened at another retreat she attended. A suggestion was made that anyone who felt that he or she had been reincarnated from the Holocaust should meet in a certain place. At least thirty people showed up. Another woman overheard our conversation and said that she too believed that she had been reincarnated from the Holocaust. She said that the poor, tormented soul who had been murdered was rewarded with her life, which has been remarkably stress-free.

A woman wearing a dress with a bright floral pattern was sitting on the floor near me. It was she who had spoken so movingly at breakfast about her murdered grandmother. The woman read aloud a poem she had written after lunch. It concerned her grandmother, whose spirit had risen within her during the morning service. The poem recreated a Shabbos in pre-war Vilna when her grandmother was surrounded by family and friends and the spirit of God blessed their Shabbos meal. As she spoke, I felt the spirit of my beloved grandmother, dead for eighteen years now, rising within me too.

On Sunday morning after breakfast, Paula and Josephine, members of my synagogue in Amherst, discussed the work of the *Chevrah Kedishah*, the ritual burial society. The *Chevrah Kedishah* washes the body of a dead person, says prayers over the corpse, dresses the corpse in a shroud, puts it into a plain pine coffin, and accompanies it to the cemetery. When Paula was asked if it is a spiritual experience, she nodded her head and replied, "Oh wow, is it."

The woman who had read the poem about her grandmother raised her hand and told the story of her grandmother's shroud. Her grandmother had kept a shroud for her own funeral, but there were many poor people in the area of Vilna where she lived. Each time a poor person died, the grandmother gave her shroud to the poor person's family and made a new one for herself. She kept doing this for years. Then the Nazis came. They marched a group of Jews including the grandmother and her mother, the speaker's great-grandmother, to the pits of Ponary on the outskirts of town, forced them to undress, shot them both in the head, and buried them naked in a mass grave. Her voice trembling, the woman said that her grandmother had never been buried in her own shroud. Then she turned to Paula and said, "The next time you wash a dead woman's corpse, think of it as my grandmother's corpse. Finally she will have a proper Jewish burial."

I was stunned, as was everyone else. It was another moment of deep connectedness, of which this retreat offered many. The woman and Paula hugged each other for five minutes or more. In May 2003 my son Michael and I would visit the pits of Ponary, where tens of thousands of our people had been murdered. As we stood there and listened to a freight train lumbering by, I said a prayer for this woman's grandmother and great-grandmother and all the other victims who had been murdered here.

After lunch I spoke with Danielle, the woman who had fallen asleep and snored at the Friday night service. I mentioned that one of the most powerful lessons of this retreat was the confirmation that *am Yisrael chai*, that the nation of Israel lives. Danielle said that she had a story to tell me. While returning to the US from a trip to Israel, she recently spent a few days in Rome.

"I know how the story ends," I said.

She stared at me.

"You're going to tell me about the Arch of Titus, right?" Danielle slowly nodded her head. The arch depicts the destruction of the Second Temple and the Jews being led off as slaves. "Inside the arch," I said, "someone has scrawled the Hebrew words *am Yisrael chai*. The power and glory of ancient Rome are gone, but we're still here."

When in amazement Danielle asked how I knew, I replied that this retreat had given me mind-reading powers. Actually, a Jewish friend who recently visited Rome told me the same story, but I didn't reveal that to Danielle.

As I was pulling out of the parking lot of the Buddhist Center to go home, I saw the woman who had told the story about her grandmother's shroud. I got out of my car and walked up to her. We had already hugged after she had read her poem. I hugged her again and whispered, "I don't even know your name, and yet I feel that I know you well." I then asked why her grandmother had stayed in Europe rather than come to America. Shirley thought that it was because someone in the family had typhus, but she didn't know for sure.

I then climbed back into my car, drove slowly down the dirt road, and without looking back, headed home. Nothing was on my mind as the universe was breathing through me, my breath, Shirley's breath, God's breath. *Am Yisrael,* the nation of Israel was living through us. Truly we are breathed. Truly we are lived.

When I got home after the hour ride, Alison greeted me with a lovely lunch and told me about her weekend. A pile of mail was sitting on my desk. The manuscript of my math book was open to the chapter on which I had been working. Michael needed help with his homework, and there was a problem with the computer. A few days later, I started to record my memories of the retreat, praying that I could capture my precise emotions at the moment I realized that I was being breathed and being lived by the universe, by God, by the source of all breath. I wanted to freeze these emotions, milk them, cherish them, and frame them for eternity.

But by the time I wrote it, the experience had become the shadow of a memory. I then realized, to my horror, that I was no longer being breathed. I was no longer being lived. Having already detached itself from *am Yisrael,* my ego resumed its eternal struggle against all the other suffering egos that peopled the planet. Its biggest regret was the long weekend it had lost while I was meditating in Barre and singing Shabbos songs.

❖ ❖ ❖

More than one hundred months passed, and my world changed.

On a Saturday in August 2003, I returned to Barre to participate in an eight-day retreat, encouraged to attend by Jean Colucci. Hopeful because of the auspicious signs, I vowed that this time would be different. I had been meditating regularly for half a year, my therapy with Jean was going well, and the headaches during the past few weeks had not been bad. Having made so much progress while meditating forty-five minutes a day, I was eager to see what eight days of immersion would do. This would be the crown on my sabbatical semester, the sabbatical within the sabbatical. Just to be safe, I was arriving at the retreat early. In case the room I was assigned was not perfect, I would be able to change it.

Despite my expectations, the experience of the retreat would be nothing that I could have imagined. Soon after it started, I found myself plunging into the Grand Canyon without a parachute.

The retreat was held at the Insight Meditation Society (IMS) in Barre, a short walk from the Barre Center for Buddhist Studies, where the 1994 retreat had taken place. The home of IMS is an imposing brick mansion that once housed a Christian seminary. One can find memories of the Christian past in two stained glass windows located in the room through which one walks to reach the meditation hall. The window on the right artfully and emotionally portrays an enlightened being: Jesus in vivid colors gazing up to heaven, kneeling before a rock on which his hands are folded, a halo encircling his head. The window on the left shows Jesus at a table breaking bread, a disciple or an angel leaning on Jesus in a pose of infinite respect and sadness.

Founded in 1975 "as a nonprofit organization to uphold the possibility of liberation for all beings," IMS has become a world center for the practice of moment-to-moment awareness known as insight meditation, or *vipassana* in the Buddhist tradition. When I arrived there at the earliest possible time of 3:00 PM, a man and a woman, both with German accents, signed me in. My room was A116 in the annex. My heart sank when I saw it. It was right next to a big bathroom, whose flushing toilets in the middle of the night would certainly wake me up. When I asked the retreat manager, Larry Smith, for a different room, he gladly accommodated me, giving me room A115.

Room A115 was even worse. Located in the corner of the building, it looked onto an active driveway, a door into the building, and a porch door that, like the building door, squeaked whenever it was opened, and right underneath the window there was a laundry vent. What to do? I had been here five minutes and had already fucked up. When I was in A116, I should have checked out the other rooms in the area including this one, but I didn't.

Panic. Larry was nowhere to be found. As the participants kept arriving and as the inventory of available rooms kept dwindling, I spent the next hour and a half repeatedly going back to the main office to find Larry, expecting him to be angry with me if I asked for another change. But when I found him, he wasn't angry at all. He cheerfully reassigned me to room A114 across the hall, which upon first examination seemed to be perfect. But it wasn't. Only a thin wall separated it from two other doors that slammed shut with an audible thud. Room A113 next to mine, though dangerously close to the bathroom, was probably the closest room to perfection in the annex. But I didn't have the nerve to ask again.

My adventure with the rooms was a perfect metaphor for how the mind works, trying to control and arrange the world according to its preconceived plan. I never learned whether room A113 was perfect. Although they were a little too close together, A107, A108, and A109 in the carpeted part of the annex away from the bathroom and all the doors, facing the woods in the back, were definitely the best rooms in the place. I made a note of this for the next retreat I would attend.

The leaders of the retreat were Lena Vastic and Benny Luberoff.* I had benefited from Benny's teachings in a tape called "Suffering and Pain" that a friend had lent me. He led the 8:15 sitting on Sunday morning, the first full day of the gathering. Jewish face, Jewish name. I was craving the familiar as I embarked on this journey into the unknown. All the good spots in the front of the meditation hall were occupied by participants who had been faster than I was to claim them.

At the end of the sitting Benny asked for questions. From my chair on the left side, forehead throbbing and pain threatening my nose, I asked him about chronic pain and meditation. He answered sensitively and compassionately, summarizing years of experience. Give attention to the sensation of pain, he said, but don't crowd it. Bring awareness to it but with a light touch and lots of space. Attention brings energy to a sensation, and the energy might increase the pain. So with headaches it might be better to focus on the stomach rather than on the breath.

---

* The names of the leaders of the retreat and of the retreat manager have been changed as have the dates of the retreat.

I was annoyed. Why didn't anyone ever tell me that? That one piece of advice could be more helpful than all the pills I ever took. Benny also spoke about the expectations one might have about one's pain. I had serious expectations. I wanted the facial pain to disappear forever. I came to this retreat looking for enlightenment, but in only the short time I have been here, my face hurt more than ever. What if it lasts for the rest of my life?

Lena Vastic gave a talk after the non-dinner of tea and rice cakes. I was too hungry to listen; instead, my mind began to wander. Last week our daughter Melissa had visited us, reading on a lounge chair in the backyard as she used to do when she was in high school before she met Ken and fell in love. I asked her if I could delete her files on a computer I was setting up for Alison. "Sure," she said without a thought. When I asked whether she wanted to look them over first, she laughed and replied that she hasn't needed them during the past year, so why bother?

I so admired Melissa's nonchalance. I was still unable to let her go although she was married now. Why did she have to grow up?, I asked myself as I deleted her files, thinking of the cyber-suicide I had committed last year when by mistake I deleted all the files on my office computer and had to spend half a day frantically restoring them instead of being with Melissa, who was visiting us at the time.

I fell asleep in my monastic room A114 listening to Benny's tape "Suffering and Pain."

I woke up at 3:30 AM on Monday to a disaster. My nose was throbbing with the all-day pinching pain, which, according to three years of experience and hundreds of attacks, would not go away at least until Tuesday morning 27 hours from now, no matter what I did. Despair. This was not supposed to happen. Did pushing the pain away yesterday cause this pain? Why was I staying here? The food was awful. The rice cakes, peanut butter, and fruit last night left me starved, and my fucking nose hurt like hell. I was very afraid. I wanted to go home.

I showered, probably waking up the guy in the room next to the bathroom, and then meditated. It was 6:00 AM. Should I ask to speak with Benny for a magic incantation that would make the pain disappear, like the monk's back pain in his tape? During the past week I had had no headache pain at all, and now it was a raging conflagration.

During the first sitting in the meditation hall after breakfast, a woman in the back loudly moaned and then fainted. "Is there a doctor in the house?", someone shouted. This put my suffering in perspective and emboldened me to seek out Larry Smith again. I found him in the front office and told him that this morning I had been on the verge of going home because the nose pain was not on my agenda for this retreat. He listened to me as patiently as he had yesterday when I underwent the ordeal of the multiple room-changes, and he assured me that my experiences were typical. Give it another chance, he advised.

"Do you know anything about Benny Luberoff's background?" I asked.

Larry gave me the answer I was looking for. "I think that he's Israeli."

No wonder I loved Benny's tape. I left a note for him on the bulletin board that he soon answered. "Richard, looking forward to meeting with you at 4:45. Come to room M113."

The morning unfolded more smoothly than it had begun. During the meditation sitting, I focused on the pressure of the chair against my butt and the pressure of the ground against my feet, noticing that as I brought my attention away from my face, the nose pain decreased, at times almost disappearing, exactly as Benny had promised. An amazing discovery. At the level of pure awareness without the drama, I perceived that the pressure on my nose equals the pressure of gravity on my butt equals the pressure of gravity on my feet. I don't desire that gravity disappears, so why ask the same of the nose pain? Just like gravity, I can't control it. So let it go.

After lunch I took a walk, but was bombarded with insects that tormented me every step of the way. My nose pain came roaring back, a locomotive that couldn't be stopped.

My morning insights about the pain were so obvious, yet so deep. I wanted to start my discussion with Benny by sharing them with him, but was surprised to hear myself asking whether he was Israeli. "No," he replied. "My father was Israeli, Jewish, but I grew up in Canada." Although Benny was totally compassionate with me and seemed to take great interest in the insights I had had, I perceived a thin membrane separating us. Had I offended him by my too personal question about his origin? When I was unable to answer a question he asked me, he comforted me by saying not to worry, you did not fail.

During the Monday evening sitting, I played yo-yo with my attention, focusing on my nose and feeling the pain throb, then focusing on my feet and feeling the pain ebb. Nose, feet, nose, feet, back and forth for forty-five minutes. I felt sad that Melissa got married, even though she and Ken were deeply in love. My headaches started during the preparations for her wedding. Maybe the facial pain encodes my not wanting to let her go. Why don't I let her go? I like to suffer and wallow in self-pity.

I found it effortless to bring my entire attention to brushing my teeth. When I did so, the pain disappeared. I had started the day by cursing the all-day pain. I ended the day by blessing the pain because it had led me to the insight about focusing my attention elsewhere in the body. My room was small, 8.5 by 13 feet; a chest of drawers, a sink, a bed, and a chair were all that I had. But I was starting to feel safe here.

As I fell asleep, I ran the lessons of the day through my mind. Pain is not an absolute. It's an interpretation in the mind. Not bad for a novice.

Tuesday, August 5, 2003. This was to be the day of my great breakthrough. But that wasn't obvious at 2:00 AM as I awakened from a fitful sleep. Obsessing about the headaches, the mere thought of which could make them happen, I gulped down two Tylenol PM tablets, lifesavers that always plunged me into sleep even when the pain was throbbing at its worst, but not tonight when they granted me barely two hours of rest. These headaches are huge. They're overshadowing everything. Up at 5:10. No pain at all. Joy. I lay in bed to savor it.

At the 6:00 AM sitting, I sat on my chair in the meditation hall and closed my eyes. The room was half full of tired meditators. Oh my God, slight but perceptible pain was flowing into the nose. The neuralgia beast was awake and moving. Not again. Don't want to deal with that. Very vivid sensation of my bare feet on the cold floor as the slight pain in the left nostril ebbed and flowed upward across the lower forehead. Back to my breath warily. No extra pain in my nose. Shit, here it comes again. I feel so tired. Drugged. Weary.

During the walking meditation after breakfast, deep sadness over Alison's sickness in Spain four months ago and deeper sadness over my novel and especially over Melissa. I was holding onto my nose pain as I was holding onto her, refusing to let her go. A drop of water cupped by a leaf on the side of the path gleamed in the sun. Lena Vastic's Dharma talk on Buddhist teachings last night and her story about the samurai warrior:

A samurai warrior was walking down the path while contemplating the mystery of life. He saw his teacher, a monk, sitting on the side of the path. He asked, "O master, what is heaven and what is hell?"

The monk replied, "I would not waste words on you. Your uniform is dirty, your body stinks, and your sword is dull. You are a disgrace to all samurais."

The samurai became enraged and screamed, "How dare you talk to me like that!" He pulled out his sword and ran toward the monk. When the blade was a hair's length from the monk's neck, the samurai stopped in horror and fell to the ground.

"That, my son, is hell."

The samurai understood and said, "I am deeply grateful to you, O master, for risking your life to give me this teaching." His face was radiant as he knelt down and kissed the hem of the monk's garment.

The monk said, "And this, my son, is heaven."

My father criticizing me, my father praising me. Lena's German-accented confession that she has been suffering for years with knee pain and that meditation doesn't make it better. I loved her.

During the 11:30 sitting on Tuesday a major insight bubbled up out of nowhere. My headaches have taught me so much about myself, my relationships, my life, but I was always angry at my teacher. When it comes, I might say, "Welcome. I am open to whatever you will share with me today." That is how one greets an honored teacher. Instead, I always shunned it, cursed it, pushed it away. Like my father, I protected myself. My body felt tight, constricted, controlled. Let the pain do what it wants. The truth is in my pain. The truth is in my face. Let the pain guide me, not me guide the pain. Like Alison, it has much more wisdom than I. Exactly as Jean Colucci said, cursing the pain sets up duality. Loving it makes it mine.

Melissa was funny and beautiful and smart, the fruit of my love for my darling wife, who had saved my life by opening me to love. Melissa was Alison. Just before her wedding my father accused me on the phone. . . . No, I won't go that way because he gave me my love of books and taught me math and how to write and said I should study German and drove me back to Harvard every weekend when I saw Alison but hardly spoke with him. Guilt. Sadness. Regret. Within a year he was dead, his anger turned back on himself. Losing Melissa and disagreeing with Alison about the wedding. The sadness and elation I felt when Melissa held hands with Ken during her graduation from medical school. When did that lovely child become this beautiful woman? No wonder my nerves caught on fire. Benny's attentiveness yesterday to my comment that the headaches and the wedding were connected clued me into the connection between the pain and Melissa.

I couldn't eat lunch. I sobbed on my pillow over losing Melissa and over Alison, the love of my life who is beautiful and warm, both blessed with a natural grace. While I cried over my daughter, Alison was now visiting her in New York City. My head didn't hurt. I loved my pain as I would love my best teacher. Love the pain. Don't shun the pain. Honor the pain. Don't curse the pain. The truth is in my pain. What does that mean? It will go away when it has nothing more to teach me. It will go away when I no longer need it to go away.

I have experienced such beauty in my life. I, who so wanted to control life, could not control life just as I could not control the pain, which had a mind of its own. The nature of mind. The pain was the lens through which I understood all the teachings. Loving it transcends duality, like Kafka's parable about the leopards in the temple. Make the attack of the leopards part of the ritual. Make the subversive book part of the canon, the Book of Job, the sex-drenched Song of Songs, Ecclesiastes, Lamentations. Make the random noise that disturbs my meditation part of the meditation. It was all a matter of where one put the boundary defining the ego-membrane between I and not-I.

That evening Benny gave a beautiful Dharma talk, which touched me deeply. Speaking about vulnerability and control and fear, he read my heart. We crave certainty and fear change, but the only certainty is death. Accepting the groundlessness of our being opens the door to wisdom.

For three and a half years the truth has been in my face. Today I finally saw it. Pain, my third eye, the wisdom source in the center of my face, I honor you in your infinite mystery.

On the first day Benny had instructed us on the five precepts, which we were to follow during the entire retreat:

1. Do not kill.
2. Do not steal.
3. Do not indulge in sexual misconduct.
4. Do not make false speech.
5. Do not take intoxicants.

Back in my room at the end of my Tuesday of insights — no lock, no key, only a door separating me from the world — a mosquito buzzed in my ear, a little flying thing whizzed by, a spider hung in midair on an invisible thread. One must not deliberately kill any living creature. But I wanted to sleep, and so I stood on a chair and destroyed them all. My mind, extremely calm when I had entered the room, became agitated. I harmed myself much more than the insects would have done.

At dawn on Wednesday, before anyone else got up, I sat on the wall in front of the main building and shut my eyes. No pain at all. How delicious. No pain for ten full minutes. It's better than sex. My mind is depraved. Even when the pain wasn't there, it went looking for it. Unlike me, the mind was always successful. Slight twinges during the rest of the sitting, but ninety-nine percent pain-free, the first nearly pain-free meditation in three and a half years. I'm hung up on numbers, just like an accountant, although I tell everyone that mathematicians are not accountants.

Do not steal. Do not take what is not freely given. Accept what is offered without trying to change it in any way. On the way back to my room I celebrated the nearly pain-free meditation by taking a catalog from the book closet when no one was looking. On Saturday I changed my room twice. I was shameless.

In the meditation hall after breakfast Benny gave more instructions. Open yourselves up to all aspects of your existence — the pleasant, the unpleasant, the neutral. Savor every moment with pleasure and equanimity. Do not judge. Try not to expect anything. In this way everything will open to you.

Luxuriating in the glow of Benny's words, I shut my eyes to meditate. Wham. A torrent of pain slammed the center of my nose. Before breakfast, no pain, the first time in years. After breakfast, all-day pain. But this time I listened to it. It's me. It's my pain, my body. It's teaching me to apply the insights of yesterday. Thank you, my teacher. I honor you in your infinite wisdom as you remind me about my former unskillful existence, when conditions came together that made it possible for you to happen.

At my request, Benny agreed to meet with me privately for a second time on Wednesday afternoon. When I told him about loving my pain and putting an end to aversion and feeling the tightness in my body and how Melissa was perfect, he smiled and said, "Lovely," pointing out that not only did I have the insights, but also they opened an entire emotional landscape. He was so wise. "Richard, it is not your pain that causes suffering but the mental state associated with the pain. A goal of meditation is not to show preference for pain versus no-pain, but to accept everything with equanimity and patience."

I owed Benny a deep debt of gratitude for helping me see that the most profound truths can often be stated simply. I wanted to hug him. I wanted to ask why he couldn't have been my father. A glance at the clock on the wall made me nervous. It was 5:15, but I had to start eating by 5:15 so that I could start my daily task of washing the dinner dishes by 5:40 so that I could get to the 6:30 sitting on time. I thanked Benny for his support and his wisdom and rushed off to dinner.

It was impossible to get everything done on time. Although I gulped down the delicious lentil soup without really tasting it and although I started washing the dishes five minutes early because my partner had already started and I felt guilty letting him work alone, we didn't finish until 6:25. Should I shower and risk not being on time or should I go to the sitting with smelly underarms? Either way I would disturb people. Because I opted for the former, I walked in ten minutes late.

Benny betrayed me. Walking in just ahead of me, he turned and said, "I've noticed that you've walked late into the meditation hall several times."

I felt guilty and angry. Benny, I thought, you're walking in late too, as you've already done a number of times, in fact more than I have. And your walking in late is much more disruptive than mine because you're a leader of this retreat and one of the gurus we novices look up to, but as I now see, shouldn't. "I'm very sorry," I replied, avoiding eye contact. "I had to do the dishes and it took too long." Just yesterday, when I had been meditating alone in room M101, he barged in and insensitively announced that I would have to leave because there would be interviews in this room.

"Okay. Just walk in quietly and try not to be late again."

I was in a rage but I couldn't scream. I hated Benny, beautiful at 5:00 and beastly at 6:40. My nose throbbing, I paid no attention to Lena's talk on the ten perfections: compassion, wisdom, generosity, lovingkindness, blah-blah-blah. These Buddhists love lists. But one perfection was missing from her ten: the perfection of humor. This place was too damn serious, as were most of the people. During the group interviews they all seemed genuinely troubled, their faces etched with grief. Why was I here? What were my goals? Why wasn't I with Alison visiting Melissa in New York?

I caught the end of Lena's talk, the ten perfections having all washed together. It was a Zen saying. When my house burned down, I finally had an unobstructed view of the moonlit sky. I hated Benny, but loved her. Her Austrian accent, slightly halting speech, grey hair, the face of someone who has suffered. She has meditated for thirty years, and her knee still hurt.

Zombie-like we marched to our rooms at the end of the talk. My nose was killing me, and Benny had pissed me off. I laughed. Yes, the place was too serious, but I was buying into it. So he criticized me. Who cares? I should be flattered that he felt comfortable telling me what he did. Was he testing me?

Out of spite, out of humor, out of revenge, I decided to break another rule of the retreat. Having killed three insects, having appropriated a catalog from the book closet when no one was looking, having taken food before the gong sounded, having brought food back to my room — a real pain if it attracted insects because then each insect would have to be led safely outside without being harmed — having walked in late to several sittings, though not as many as Benny, having eaten the first lunch even though I was assigned to the second lunch, having kept a journal, and having read a book, I non-Buddhistly craved some ice cream, which wasn't a crime, but leaving IMS and driving my car into the center of town and buying the oversize strawberry ice cream cone certainly were.

Next to the ice cream place was a liquor store. Against the back wall was a life-size poster of a big-titted model spilling out of her bikini with a Bud in her hand. The nose pain vanished while I sank my tongue into the ice cream and licked it lasciviously. I circled around to get another look at the model, and the pain returned. Do not indulge in sexual misconduct, Benny had told us on the first day. I finally understood that it was for my protection. I walked past the liquor store and forced myself not to look in. A strawberry mustache on my face, I returned to my monastic cell at IMS.

I still hated Benny. Had he punished me because I offended him by my question whether he was a Jew?

At the 6:00 AM sitting on Thursday, I felt a configuration of energy shifting in my face, settling in my nose, jumping to my jaw, the nose pain lessening. Benny was right. I saw clearly that the facial pain was fluid and changeable and always wanted to move. It's energy, not mass. The tightness in the nose that happened during breakfast vanished while I was writing from

7:00 to 8:00. The handwriting in my journal has become as calm as I am.

During the 8:15 sitting the tightness returned and blossomed almost instantaneously into the pinching nose-pain that has always driven me crazy but now was losing its sting. The third time in four days, the most I've had it since the headaches had started. Why? I would never know. Give up knowing, a constriction of the consciousness that blocks the laser light of wisdom, a roof blocking the view of the moonlit sky.

More meditation instructions. More talk about consciousness and mind and factors affecting the mind. Mental states, emotions, thoughts, words tumbling over words, losing their meaning.

The days were flowing together, each one like the day before. The drama was all internal. What will come up for me today? It was so calm here that the least disturbance — rushing to eat the non-dinner in order to finish the dishes in order to get to the evening sitting on time or Benny's telling me that I was late — caused great mental agitation.

Something extraordinary happened. A vision beyond words. I was overwhelmed by emotion as I saw Melissa young, two years old in her yellow outfit, and she was calling to me, "Play with me, Dad." Then falling in love with Alison and being with her during weekends at Harvard, so happy together, and with Alison and Melissa when Alison was young and beautiful and I was young too, and with Alison and Melissa and Michael in Israel in 1982, Michael driving a piece of pita bread. Going to Jerusalem the first time and seeing the Old City and the Western Wall, overwhelmed by emotion and connection with the Jewish people. How good to be alive. And while visualizing all this, I cried. Tears of joy and happiness over the beauty of my life, even though my nose hurt. Tears of joy at this gorgeous day, which had started with me sitting on the wall outside under the huge blue sky, and while meditating, I kept repeating "spaciousness, spaciousness" and imagining that my mindscape was the huge blue sky, my bad feelings about Benny a teaspoon of salt in a fresh-water lake the size of the Milky Way. The deep gong of the bell. Sleepers, awake. The sitting was over. An altar at the front of the meditation hall with a statue of the Buddha and two vases filled with flowers. I cried. Alison — her simplicity and beauty.

I gazed out the open window. Sun, blue sky, no clouds, light breeze, 70 degrees and no humidity, birds chirping. It was September 11 again. The guy meditating ten feet away with the Jewish face and the 9/11 T-shirt: NYPD and NYFD — Gone but Not Forgotten. Alison with Melissa today while I was here. So happy they could be together. Great oceans of feeling continued to surge inside me. I had no expectations when I sat down on time at 8:15 today on my uncomfortable chair for which the cushions were never quite right — one too thick and the other too thin. The speaker was boring, and then the ocean swelled.

What was happening? The nose pain and Melissa and Alison were intimately connected in ways I would never figure out. As I accessed this vast emotional landscape within me, as I opened up to these memories of beauty and love and loss, the frozen tightness in my nose flowed. When the sitting was over, I stood by the window and felt the sun on my face. Those waves of love and beauty that had overwhelmed me were so palpable, a warm glow that spread its radiance all over me. Alison in white, Melissa in yellow, Alison and I swinging Melissa back and forth as we walked, Melissa giggling with joy. What must I let go of?

I felt connected the entire day. At 10:00 I meditated in my favorite place, the high-backed chair in room M101 that Benny had kicked me out of, a photo of the meditation teacher, Dipa Ma, on the mantle. More images of love and beauty. Melissa being born, our trip across the US in 1978. So many years together. Alison, I love you.

At 11:00 I took a walk wearing an insect net. It worked. It's just like life, where meditation was the insect net. My mind was focused. For many minutes I could follow my feet on the ground, feeling the pressure of the pavement.

At 12:15 I showered and paid attention to every aspect of it. Miraculous how my nose didn't hurt while I was in the moment, paying attention to the shower, and then the mind wandered, looking for the pain, which obligingly returned.

Thank you, great master, for revealing to me the nature of mind.

I tried it again at lunch, and it continued to work. I took a mouthful of food, shut my eyes, and concentrated, my attention focused on the food, the sensation so vivid. I was my mouth. There was no "I," only the chewing. The infinite variety: pasta salad, onions, spices, tomato salad, the infinite textures in a mouthful of sprouts, chickpeas, sunflower seeds, dressing. I could taste everything. I was everything except "I." There was no pain.

This was the purpose of the teaching. If I hadn't had the pain in my nose today, I wouldn't have been able to experience the disappearance of the pain when I showered or ate or shitted or brushed my teeth. Thank you, pain, for teaching me again. Thank you for teaching me about the nature of monkey mind, which was to follow old patterns, to look for the pain as soon as the attention wandered and to find the pain. I finally understood the meaning of letting go. It meant to stop looking for it. When I realized this, I cried again, feeling no shame because I loved these people for their silence and for letting me cry. One thin guy with a wispy beard and a face that looked really weird when he did walking meditation picked up a spider from the floor of the meditation hall, cupped it in his hand, walked to the window, lifted the screen, and released it.

In the late afternoon on Thursday, I meditated again in room M101. As I was walking back to the stairs, a woman emerged from the bathroom. Through the closed door I had heard her coughing and retching. We made eye contact, and I stopped to let her go before me. When we reached the bottom of the stairs, she turned, looked at me, joined her palms at chest level in the Buddhist gesture of gratitude, bowed, and smiled a most beautiful smile. Alison's smile.

Poor Sheldon was gone. Tall, overweight, the model of a New York Jew with greasy hair, always agitated, constantly writing in his room with the door open. On Sunday, when Benny had invited questions about the experience of meditation, Sheldon asked about the conceptual differences between Buddhism and Taoism. Today at breakfast he cut to the head of the line, breaking the silence of the retreat by saying that he's on dishwashing duty. The woman next to me smiled.

Lena Vastic was a beautiful person, warm and lovable. Her Dharma talk on Thursday was on equanimity, *Gleichmut* in German. A beautiful word. Deeply conditioned patterns of reactivity make us crave the pleasant and reject the unpleasant. Lena possessed the eleventh perfection of humor, speaking about the laughter of wisdom, the laughter of letting go. With great compassion, Lena explained the difficulty of attaining equanimity:

> "If you can accept all of life's failures in the same way you accept the successes, if you have no jealousy when your neighbor buys a new car or takes a wonderful trip, if you can happily accept

whatever food is put on your plate, if after a busy day of running around you can fall asleep without a drink or a pill," — Lena took a deep breath and surveyed the audience — "then you are a dog."

She brought the house down, the funniest line of the retreat.

After Lena's talk, I followed her unspoken advice by driving into town and buying a mint chocolate chip ice cream cone smothered in Heath Bar Crunch. I tasted every bite. When I went to bed at 9:50, my nose was hurting badly.

I woke up early on Friday morning and meditated in my room. Insight after insight came upon me, ocean waves of wisdom in which I swimmingly luxuriated. To always live life as open as I was at that moment. Do I wish that or do I fear that? Melissa being born, me changing her diapers — tears came to my eyes as I wrote this in my room because it went deep — me playing with her as a kid, Melissa playing with the dollhouse my father had made for her, his supreme act of love. Suffering arises from clinging, so let it go. But it kept on coming, my entire life in vivid, kaleidoscopic detail, wave after wave. This is how the mind works. I should have spent more time with Melissa when she was young, as Alison did. "Mommy, what can we do together now?" On Mother's Day Melissa had sent Alison a card saying, "You are my best friend." I cried as I wrote this in my room, and I cry as I transcribe it now. This was what it meant to let go of Melissa. It meant letting go of the opportunities I might have missed. I had done my best and had not failed.

Like the pain, insight and wisdom bubbled up into consciousness of their own accord and without my intervention.

Then the insight and the wisdom hit a wall. The participants in the retreat had been divided into small groups that were to meet with each of the leaders in a group interview. The interview with Benny was scheduled for 3:00. I was dreading it because of his outrageous behavior on Wednesday when he scolded me for being late at the evening sitting because I had washed my underarms after washing the dinner dishes. Despite my dread, I showed up at the assigned room on time, not looking at Benny because, as I realized at that moment, I hated him.

Benny instructed us to talk about our current feelings concerning the retreat or our meditation practice.

I would be the second person to speak. The band of pain slicing my eyes got tighter. While waiting for my turn, I carefully rehearsed what I would say. On Monday I woke up with a bad headache, the breakfast was lousy, and I craved a lobster and a cold beer. I was very close to packing up and going home. But I stayed, and yesterday I was rewarded for staying. I would then talk about the feelings of love and connection with my wife and children that welled up within me and the memories of our life together that enveloped me, followed by. . . .

Without warning I heard my name. "Richard, what would you like to tell us?"

I felt the words start to roll glibly off my tongue. "On Monday, I woke up with a bad headache, the breakfast was. . . ."

Benny cut me off. "Today is Friday. We already discussed what happened on Monday."

Without missing a beat, I jumped to the present. "I find myself totally in the moment. When I shower, I am mindful of every motion of my hands. When I eat, I am mindful of every bite, and I taste all the exquisite, intricate textures of the food. The practice has really paid off. While showering mindfully and while eating mindfully, the pain in my head completely disappears." Then looking deeply into Benny's eyes, I added, "I want to thank you for all your help and guidance this week." In spite of everything, I loved him again.

His eyes shimmering, he looked back at me with gratitude and love. "Thank you."

I have played this scene over and over again hundreds of times. After he rudely interrupted me, reminding me that we had already discussed what happened on Monday, why didn't I stay silent? Why didn't I storm out of the room, making a scene? Why didn't I shout, "Fuck you, Benny. Get off my back."? I didn't stay silent and I didn't storm out and I didn't shout because I was in the moment, and the moment was all I had. Despite my dread, the interview ended up being the ultimate test of mindfulness and of being in the moment and thus the ultimate test of the teachings. How fortunate I was that the pain had opened me up to them.

While I was waiting in line for dinner that evening, a young woman, a teenager perhaps, walked with a small flower vase outside. Blue top, white shorts, innocent and peaceful smile, she was carrying a bunch of flowers, mostly daisies and some larger red flowers. She bent down and in a gesture of infinite beauty cut another flower for her bouquet. Melissa carrying flowers as a child. Thank you, my child, for bringing such beauty into my life. As I lay in bed in my room that night, it was raining gently. The sound of the rain falling through the trees just outside my window was so peaceful. Time to rest.

The final lunch of the retreat was a sensual delight. Barbecued tofu with a tangy sauce, brown basmati rice, cauliflower, broccoli, carrots, lettuce, sprouts, raisins, chickpeas, sunflower seeds, dressing, chocolate-chip oatmeal bars. I took small amounts into my mouth and savored everything. Again there was no "I"; there was only eating.

Time to go home. Time to say goodbye to this refuge of my awakening. Time to say goodbye to Benny, who was not at the door waiting to apologize to me. Time to let him go. Time to let it all go. Trying to capture the insights of these eight days was like trying to capture the sunset. Life is a spiritual journey home to the place we've always been because the wisdom of our Buddha nature is within us and does not have to be learned. To discover the elephant of wisdom in our hearts, we only have to remove everything that is not-elephant.

When I got home, I looked at our house in wonder. Here is where we raised our two beautiful children. The red flowers that Alison had planted in the front yard were on fire. The green of the trees was pulsing. I felt truly blessed.

Alison's car was gone. She had expressed her Buddha nature by arranging on the kitchen table the photos from her five days in New York City with Melissa.

> Dear Rich,
> Welcome home! Sure did miss you. Had to get some grub. Look at photos from NYC. Fabulous time. Hope you did too. I love you.
> Alison

The truth is in my face. The wisdom of Kalu Rinpoche, the great Tibetan master, was confirmed once again by the insights that the pain had granted me during the retreat in Barre:

> This ability to recognize the open, empty nature of mind and all its productions, projections, thoughts, and emotions is the panacea, the

universal remedy that in and of itself cures all delusion, all negative emotion, and all suffering.

Our mind can be compared to a hand that is bound or tied up, as much by the representation of our "me," of the ego or self, as by the conceptions and fixations belonging to this idea. Little by little, Dharma practice eliminates these self-cherishing fixations and conceptions, and, just as an unbound hand can open, the mind opens and gains all kinds of possibilities for activity. It then discovers many qualities and skills, like the hand freed from its ties. The qualities that are slowly revealed are those of enlightenment, of pure mind.

Mindfulness is this ability to recognize the open, empty nature of mind and all its productions, projections, thoughts, and emotions. It is the universal solvent for all negative mindstates. It is love and lovingkindness directed to ourselves and through ourselves, to the entire world. As Jean Colucci taught me and as the pain constantly validates, it is the only path to deep and abiding happiness.

Before Alison returned home, I did walking meditation in the back yard of our house. The sensuality of walking barefoot on the grass, feeling the warm spots in the sun and the cool spots in the shade. A butterfly with beautifully patterned wings fluttered from one blade to another. The sun shone on my face. The sky was a deep blue. There was a cool breeze. This, my son, is heaven.

4

Face to Face with Jacob

> And not for naught did the Gaon of Vilna tell the translator of Euclid's geometry into Hebrew [R. Barukh of Shklov], that "To the degree that a man is lacking in the wisdom of mathematics he will lack one hundredfold in the wisdom of the Torah."
> — Rabbi Joseph B. Soloveitchik, *Halakhic Man*

THE RETREAT AT THE Insight Meditation Society opened my heart to the infinite love that connects me with Alison, Melissa, Michael, my extended family, my friends, all human beings, all living beings, the universe. I wish I could say that my heart never closed again. That after the retreat the headaches disappeared and my ego became as light as a breath. It was not so. My heart continued to open and close to its own rhythms, and tugged like the tides by the sun and the moon of my unknowing, the headaches continued to flow and surge and vanish and return as I passed into and out of enlightenment, my ego as light as a breath and then with my next breath as ponderous as the planet.

But something earthshakingly fundamental had changed, and I knew it. After four decades of a spiritual search riven by duality, driven by the blessing/curse of creativity and the love/hatred of mathematics and the passion for/repulsion from Judaism, an unknowable force had guided me to that meditation center, just an hour from my home, where the innate wisdom locked within me was somehow released and was allowed to grow.

I had come to the retreat with an agenda. The facial pain must vanish forever. Then through no effort of my own I experienced the truth that is in my pain, the truth that had been in my face since February 2000. It's not the pain that causes suffering, but the mental state associated with the pain. The mystery of this wisdom. It had taken me three and a half years to understand deeply what I could now express in a single, short sentence. The mystery of this wisdom blessed me only because of the headaches, and it would eventually become an all-encompassing, artful approach to my entire life. Headaches, you are my beloved teacher. I honor you for bringing me through that desiccated landscape painted with pain to this oasis of peace. What will you teach me today?

You have already taught me that Richard S. Ellis is not the victim of the pain and is not suffering from the pain. "Richard S. Ellis" is a concept that freezes reality, violating the universal law of impermanence and change by giving the illusion of a fixed, stable identity. Within this concept there swarms a multitude of I's, their transformations occurring through no effort of any of the Richard S. Ellises with whom these I's have been labeled. As Frederick Franck concludes in his memoir, *Fingers Pointing Toward the Sacred: A Twentieth Century Pilgrimage on the Eastern and Western Way*, the pronoun "he" seems to be much more appropriate in describing this "sequence of incarnations":

Making up a provisional accounting, I was astounded to discover that I did not choose the content of a single one of these lives that form my life. In retrospect, many of their episodes seem to have happened to someone else, someone long dead, almost forgotten, someone with whom my present "I" seems to have so little in common that I am inclined to think in terms of "he" rather than "I."

It looks as if all that I ever planned or strove for had come to naught. What succeeded just happened.

A multitude of I's. "Richard S. Ellis" is nothing more than a convenient label whose many I's and many lives are transient — a rainbow, a flash of lightning, the reflection of the moon in water, the energy flow in my face. But the wisdom that has animated these lives is real.

It is the wisdom of Buddhist teachings made accessible through the headache pain. It is also the wisdom of the Hebrew Bible and mathematics, neither of which is what it seems to be. The Hebrew Bible is the bedrock text of our civilization, yet it is read almost exclusively in translation and not in the original Hebrew. This fundamental conceptual lens, often unappreciated and often misunderstood, is our civilization's greatest hidden text. Likewise, mathematics is our greatest hidden language — in the words of Galileo, "the language with which God has written the universe." This fundamental conceptual lens is the Judaism of science, as unappreciated and misunderstood as the Hebrew Bible in its original language.

My goal is not to bemoan the popular opinion of the Hebrew Bible, but to celebrate its beauty, interpretive power, and deep connection with Buddhist teachings. Our discussion will focus on the life of Jacob, the story of creation, the Garden of Eden narrative, and the Book of Job. As much as possible, we will read the text with a sensitivity to the original Hebrew. Because this experience will be new for many readers, a gentle introduction will be given. Bringing this sensitivity to the text, one sees that in many places the Hebrew of the Bible is a Buddhist language that goes beyond words and concepts, a textual analog of the Buddhist way of living that exhibits a fertile ambiguity, a fluidity of word, theme, and character pregnant with possibilities and unavailable in any translation. As we become aware of the open-endedness, multiple interpretability, and vast reach of the original Hebrew, we are inspired to bring to our daily experiences the same awareness of interdependence and infinite possibilities.

In this way, reading the Hebrew Bible Jewish-Buddhistly could be much more than an intellectual exercise. The insights that it reveals could change your life. It is a flow in which you swim, not a problem that you must solve.

Reading the Hebrew Bible with a sensitivity to its original language will highlight the treasures that have made this book, even in translation, our sacred guide and our reservoir of collective memory. Each Biblical reference evokes a complex web of associations: the serpent in the Garden of Eden, Noah's ark, the banishment from Eden, Jacob's ladder, Joseph's coat of many colors, the golden calf. Biblical references immeasurably enrich our experiences by endowing them with a spiritual history and a sacred resonance. The potency and naturalness of these references invite us to explore further the Hebrew Bible's interpretive power.

We can experience this power by using the Hebrew Bible as a conceptual lens to interpret our own lives and ultimately to change them. The story of Jacob nicely illustrates this.

A key event in Jacob's life, one of the fulcrums on which the lever of his history turns, occurs in chapter 27 of Genesis. There he took the blessing that his father Isaac had intended for his twin elder brother Esau. Jacob's deceit against his brother mirrors, in the sacred mythology of our people, the familial deceit that forever separated my grandfather from his brother in Poland. In 1923, when my grandparents and my mother, then five months old, immigrated to the US, my grandfather's brother Shulem was unable to join them. In the story told me by my Israeli relatives, his identification papers had been taken by a cousin in order to avoid being drafted into the Polish army. Instead, Shulem immigrated to Argentina, coming to Israel with his son Yosef in 1952. One of my most profound experiences was meeting Yosef, his wife Yehudit, and their family while I lived in Jerusalem in 1986.

Seething with resentment against his brother, Esau vowed to kill him. Jacob escaped, slept on a pillow of stone, and dreamed about a ladder, above which stood the LORD. Jacob's words upon awakening from his dream describe my awakening from the nightmare of the headaches. "Indeed the LORD is in this place, and I did not know" (Gen. 28:16). This place, I finally realized after years of suffering from headache pain, was my face. My face was the place where I learned the truth of my pain and where God breathed me in Barre, Massachusetts. How awe-inspiring is this place, which are the words spoken by Jacob in the next verse.

As Jacob was about to meet his brother after twenty years in exile, he wrestled with an unknown adversary on the bank of the Yabboq River. When Jacob asked the adversary for his name, the adversary refused, conveying to Jacob a basic teaching. As in life, names in the Hebrew Bible are concepts that freeze experience, violating the universal law of impermanence and change by giving the illusion of a fixed, stable identity. For Jacob, letting go of names was letting go of the past. Doing so prepared him for the face-to-face encounter with his brother, which he executed elegantly and simply. As Jacob focused on names and concepts, so did I. Not understanding that pain is a concept, I congealed it into a solid, substantial reality and then suffered from that solidification. Meditation showed me the path to peace by revealing that the pain is impermanent, continually flowing and changing. Facing the truth that is in my face, I let go of the pain, let go of the past, and finally woke up.

Jacob's story is a story of transformation: how a person focused on achievement and control discovers a new way of being, based on insight and love. Through Jacob's transformation I view my own. Through my own I view Jacob's.

Because of these interconnections with my life and other interconnections with yours, Jacob is certainly worth exploring further. Reading him with a sensitivity to the original Hebrew reveals insights, completely inaccessible in translation, into his personality and into the nature of the language in which he lives and breathes.

Jacob, in Hebrew *Yaaqov*, renamed the eponymic *Yisrael* after his fight with the unknown adversary on the banks of the anagrammatic *Yabboq* River, is the most complex of the Biblical patriarchs. He is a mosaic of his dominating, dynamic, dexterous grandfather Abraham, an attractive/repellent father-figure if there ever was one, and his contemplative, almost hidden Buddha-father Isaac. In chapter 22 of Genesis Isaac walked next to his father to the summit of Mount Moriah, where his father was intending to sacrifice him in response to God's monstrous command. Isaac, the epitome of goodness, purity, and trust, then disappears from the text, not returning until Genesis 24:63. There we watch Isaac going out to meditate in the field toward evening as Rebecca, his future wife, approached amidst a caravan of camels. In the words of Rashi, the preeminent commentator on the Hebrew Bible, when Rebecca first gazed on Isaac, she saw his goodness and purity and was astonished at the sight.*

In this dysfunctional family haunted by the near-sacrifice of the father by the grandfather, Jacob became a poet. When I read his story, I imagine that he wrote it.

A mosaic of his father and his grandfather, Jacob epitomizes the clever Jew who succeeds by his wit and guile. He is a representative of Hermes, the god of tricksters, commerce, land travel, gymnastics, and oratory known for his cunning, mercuriality, eloquence, and shrewdness. In his book, *The Jewish Century*, Yuri Slezkine observes that as an embodiment of that Greek god, Jacob "cross[es] conceptual and communal borders as a matter of course." The experiences of Jacob's life encouraged him to embrace the Hermes-qualities of flow, nonrigidity, and openness, the very qualities we want to bring to reading the Hebrew Bible. This approach is a Buddhist one. It recognizes that meaning in the Hebrew Bible is not an absolute quality of the text alone, but rather is the fruit of the reader's interaction with it. The meaning that the reader finds in the text changes as the reader's experiences change.

Jacob's story is also one of the most artful representations in the Hebrew Bible of its main theme: the entry into human

---

* All insights of Rashi concerning the Book of Genesis are taken from two translations of his commentary by Rabbi Avrohom Davis and Rabbi Meir Zlotowitz. Rashi is the acronym for Rabbi Solomon ben Isaac (1040–1105).

history of the infinite, indefinable, beyond-all-words God, who, as mourners recite in the prayer known as the Mourner's Kaddish, is above all blessings and hymns and praises and consolations that are uttered in this world (translation by Leon Wieseltier). A negative formulation of the same insight: if God could be understood through concepts, if God's existence could be mathematically proved, then it would not be God. Thus we confront the basic paradox at the heart of the Hebrew Bible's narrative art. How can words express the encounter between humans and God, who is beyond all words?

As we will see, the Hebrew language of the Bible is different from other human discourse, an ideal medium to describe the indescribability of the human-Divine encounter. If we are quiet and aware, then we can view infinite possibilities in the holy text that bridges the abyss separating God from humans. In his book on the Jacob story, *God Was in This Place and I, i Did Not Know*, Rabbi Lawrence Kushner describes the depth of the text:

> [T]he biblical word conceals an infinity of meanings. . . . We read the Bible, fix our attention on a phrase, and suddenly find ourselves in a conversation with centuries of teachers who also have come hoping to penetrate the meaning of the same text, convinced that holy words are intimately related not only to what God means but even to who God is and who we are.

Let us strive to have a creative, loving, intimate relationship with this sacred text that teaches us about ourselves. Let us strive to read the Hebrew Bible in the way that the Buddha teaches us to live: by being a verb and not a noun, a jazz riff and not a symphony; by being open to nuance and surprise and change; by not investing words and experiences with fixed meanings, but by recognizing that they are empty, a Buddhist concept conveying not a meaningless void, but a dynamic, interconnected web of significance devoid of any defining essence and therefore, like the words of the Hebrew Bible, pregnant with possibility; by wrestling with the text as Jacob wrestled with the nameless adversary at the Yabboq River; by splintering the text into sparks of new meanings by listening with an open heart and an awakened mind to the traces of God's breath within and without and between the words.

Above all, one should avoid forcing a coherent narrative on the Hebrew Bible. In doing so, one commits what Robert Alter, Bible scholar and translator of the Five Books of Moses, calls the "heresy of explanation":

> The unacknowledged heresy underlying most modern English versions of the Bible is the use of translation as a vehicle for *explaining* the Bible instead of representing it in another language, and in the most egregious instances this amounts to explaining away the Bible. This impulse may be attributed . . . to a feeling that the Bible, because of its canonical status, has to be made accessible — indeed, transparent — to all.

We can't force a coherent narrative on our lives, so why do it with the Hebrew Bible? Let the text flourish in its ambiguity and its multiple interpretability and its occasional incoherence. As we play Jewish-Buddhistly with the text of the holy Hebrew Bible, we become God's partners.

The holiness of the Hebrew Bible emanates from the language in which it is written. It is unlike any other language that you have experienced. We will start with the letters and then rise up to words, verses, and beyond.

Hebrew is a Semitic language, a close relative of Arabic and Aramaic, which Sarah and Abraham spoke before they immigrated to the land of Canaan. As Mark Oaknin explains in his book, *Mysteries of the Alphabet: The Origins of Writing*, Aramaic was the source of the form of the square-script letters of modern Hebrew. It is written from right to left, and its alphabet consists of twenty-two letters representing only consonants. The indication of vowels by adding points to the consonants came much later, well after the time when the Hebrew Bible was written.

The Hebrew alphabet developed from proto-Sinaitic, the world's first alphabet dating from the middle of the second millennium BCE, which roughly corresponds to the Exodus from Egypt and the giving of the Torah on Mount Sinai. This near synchronism is not mere coincidence. The first act of writing recorded in the Torah is God's inscribing the Ten Commandments on the dual tablets that God made and Moses smashed when the people of Israel committed the sin of the golden calf.

Like Jacob himself, each of the letters has a multiple identity, bridging the concreteness of Egyptian hieroglyphics, from which they derived, and the abstractness of Greek letters, into which they developed. First, each of the Hebrew letters represents a sound. Second, each has a numerical value corresponding to its position in the alphabet. Third, the names of most of the letters represent objects, which in turn often correspond to the forms of the letters. As one can see in the first two letters, *aleph* and *bet*, this multiple identity gives rise to fascinating, often deeply spiritual interconnections that are completely absent in the abstract alphabets of Western languages.

The letter *aleph* has no sound. It's a breath, a pause. Silence. It is the first letter of the Hebrew word *eyn*, meaning "nothingness" or "emptiness." It was honored by God by being chosen as the first letter of the first word, *anochi*, of the first of the Ten Commandments, God's in-breath before God spoke the law to Israel at Mount Sinai. Gershom Scholem, the great scholar of Jewish mysticism, explains why *aleph* may be "regarded . . . as the spiritual root of all the other letters":

> In Rabbi Mendel's view . . . [a]ll that Israel heard was the *aleph* with which in the Hebrew text the first Commandment begins, the *aleph* of the word *anokhi* [sic], "I." This strikes me as a highly remarkable statement, providing much food for thought. For in Hebrew the consonant *aleph* represents nothing more than the position taken by the larynx when a word begins with a vowel. Thus the *aleph* may be said to denote the source of all articulate sound, and indeed the Kabbalists always regarded it as the spiritual root of all the other letters, encompassing in its essence the whole alphabet and hence all other elements of human discourse.

Aleph combines the mystical and the mundane. The written form of this letter derives not from the silence on Mount Sinai, but from the fields that bring forth God's bounty. *Aleph*, meaning "ox," is written א, a skewed view of an ox's face, one horn pointing up toward the heavens, the other horn pointing down toward earth. Infinity and unity in the same symbol: adopted by the mathematician Georg Cantor to represent infinity in his theory of infinite sets, א has a numerical value of 1 signifying the interconnected unity of the infinite levels of existence, everything in the heavens and the earth and above and between and beneath, everything a manifestation of God's presence.

The second letter in the Hebrew alphabet is *bet*, which has the sound b. This letter was honored by God by being chosen as the first letter of the Hebrew Bible in the word *bereyshit*. Translated simply as "in the beginning," this word contains, as we will see in next chapter, the fractal mystery of creation embedded within it. The letter *bet* has a numerical value of 2 and, as we will also explore in the next chapter, embodies the duality principle underlying creation. Meaning "house," *bet* is written ב . It is a dwelling, a tent perhaps, with one wall open to the world.

The twenty-two letters of the Hebrew alphabet are the atoms of creation. They combine to form the word-molecules of the Hebrew Bible's sublime narrative and poetic art, an art that remains hidden from most readers because the Hebrew Bible is known intimately only through translation: the Septuagint Greek, the most fundamental of the translations because of its strong influence on all later ones; Jerome's Latin Vulgate; Luther's German Bible; the King James Bible. However, the Hebrew Bible cannot be understood when confronted through the veil of translation. Only when one confronts the text face to face in its original form can one appreciate that the Hebrew language is an ideal medium to express the richly evocative and multifaceted visions of the human-Divine encounter that are at the heart of its artistry and mystery.

Literary techniques such as paradox and wordplay flow naturally from the structure of the Hebrew language, which is based on three-letter consonantal roots. For example, consider the Hebrew noun *shalom*, meaning "peace." When written in English characters, this word has the three-letter consonantal root *sh-l-m*, which it shares with a number of words, including the adjective *shalem*, meaning "whole" or "unharmed," the noun *shlemut*, meaning "perfection," and the verb *nishlam*, meaning "it was completed." Through the transformations of its root, the meaning of a word can change radically. Here is an example involving the verb "break," taken from the novel, *The Genizah at the House of Shepher*, by Tamar Yellin. "A word begins from a root, a mere three letters, and grows like a plant through seven constructs: I break, I smash, I am broken, I am smashed, I make shatter, I am caused to break down, I devastate myself."

In its original format the Torah, comprising the Five Books of Moses, is a handwritten scroll containing only consonants but no vowels and no punctuation. As a result the reader is free — in fact, is empowered and urged — to experiment with alternate choices of vowels and punctuation marks in order to discover new meanings. Such rereadings are inevitably lost in translation, which almost always must select a single interpretation.

As we will see in a number of examples, different choices of vowels in a consonantal root in the Hebrew Bible often yield multiple meanings that immeasurably deepen the plain sense of the text. As George Steiner, the eminent writer and literary thinker, observes in his essay titled "An Introduction to the Hebrew Bible," this feature of Biblical Hebrew confers upon it a unique poetic power:

> The consonantal structure of all Hebrew writing — numerous words grow out of a radical of three consonants — is crucial. It allows, indeed

makes unavoidable, a polysemic plurality and richness of possible readings probably unmatched by any other written tongue. The same consonantal cluster can, with different vocalizations, be interpreted in wholly different senses. The omission of vowel markers generates an inherent manifold of putative meanings, of implicit puns and word-play within the identical consonantal unit. A biblical word pulses, so to speak, within an aura of concentric significations and echoes.

This insight is basic to understanding how the Hebrew Bible can speak a Buddhist language that goes beyond words. Because of the nature of Biblical Hebrew, the infinitely creative text of the Hebrew Bible is effortlessly able to generate multiple meanings, thus allowing the text to speak in multiple voices from multiple perspectives.

The lack of vowels and punctuation is but one source of the fertile ambiguity of the Hebrew Bible. The philosopher Spinoza, born Jewish but excommunicated from Judaism because of his heretical views, cites the following additional sources: the loss of meaning of numerous words after the Biblical period due to Hebrew's ceasing to be a living language; the lack of precise knowledge of Hebrew phraseology; the multiple meanings of its conjunctions and adverbs; the fact that Hebrew verbs lack a number of tenses often used in other languages; and the existence of groupings of letters having similar forms or similar sounds, resulting in errors by scribes, who in mistaking a letter for a similar one altered the text. All of these contribute to the open-endedness of the Hebrew Bible, inviting us to interpret and to create meaning by experimenting with alternate choices of vowels, punctuation marks, letters having similar shapes and sounds, and the like. We will follow this approach as we read a number of texts in Genesis and the Book of Job in this and the next two chapters.

In many printed editions of the Hebrew Bible the words have vowels and the punctuation is given. In their book on Biblical Hebrew syntax, Bruce K. Waltke and M. O'Connor explain that the vowels and the punctuation are based on the Masoretic text, which is derived from a body of scribal notes that were compiled from about 600 to 1000 CE and form a textual guide to the Hebrew Bible. Presumably an impetus for this work was the danger that the vowelless, unpunctuated text would become corrupted or would be mispronounced while being read aloud. Interestingly the stabilized Masoretic text enabled the creative genius of the Rabbinic commentators to flourish and empowers us, the readers, to become their partners in interpretation.

This is the legacy of the great Rabbinic commentators: the open-ended approach to the Hebrew Bible that hears the text speak in multiple voices from multiple perspectives. The text is ancient, but their interpretive methods are strikingly modern, as Phyllis Trible points out in her essay titled "What God Meant to Say . . .":

> To those acquainted with the wiles of deconstruction, these ancient hermeneutical maneuvers appear eerily contemporary. They witness to the indeterminacy of language, the fallacy of objectivity, the propensity for multiple reading and the desire to negotiate meanings.

In this spirit, let us now enter the ancient-modern text. We start with the story of Jacob, which is energized by a rich and intricate wordplay and by deep Buddhist insights. The unpredictability and creativity of the transformations of Jacob's name mirror the potential for creative change in Jacob's character, each transformation corresponding to a crucial episode in his life.

Jacob was born with a double curse: the curse of being double and the curse of not letting go. Rivalry and contention marked his life from conception as he and his twin brother, Esau, wrestled within their mother's womb. Esau was born first. At birth Jacob was given his Hebrew name, *Yaaqov*, because his hand was grasping Esau's heel, *Yaaqov* and the word for "heel" being connected by a common root (Gen. 25:26). Grasping and not letting go would become one of Jacob's characteristic gestures. It foreshadows not only Jacob's relationship with his double sibling, but also his relationship with life, which Jacob wanted desperately to control but which would unfold in ways he could not imagine. Until the wrestling match with the nameless adversary seven chapters later, Jacob, the Esau-grasper and the grasper of life, would not let go.

"And the lads grew up, and Esau was a man skilled in hunting, a man of the field, and Jacob was a simple man, a dweller in tents" (Gen. 25:27). Jacob the poet deceives us by this self-description as simple. When Esau returned home one day famished from the hunt, he allowed himself to be trapped by Jacob into making a lopsided exchange that had far-reaching consequences: he sold his birthright for a pot of stew that Jacob had prepared and Esau craved.

In Hebrew, "birthright" is *bechorah*, an anagram of *brachah*, which means "blessing" and was Jacob's next target. Helped by his mother and empowered by the birthright he had bought from his brother, smooth-skinned Jacob posed as hairy Esau in order to take the blessing that his blind father Isaac had intended for

Esau, his elder son. Embittered over the loss of the blessing that his father had promised him, Esau double-punned on both his double-dealing brother's name and his own double loss when he asked, "Was his name called Jacob/*Yaaqov* that he should trip me now twice by the heels/*va-yaaqveni?* My birthright/*bechorah* he took, and look, now, he's taken my blessing/*brachah*" (Gen. 27:36). As Robert Alter notes, Jacob's Hebrew name, *Yaaqov*, etymologized as "heel-grasper," is now transformed into the verb *va-yaaqveni* having the root *aqob*, meaning "crooked" and denoting devious or deceitful dealing. The heel-grasper became the heel-sneak.

Did Jacob dupe his father into giving the blessing to the wrong son? The text is silent, inviting the reader to decide on the motivations of Jacob and Isaac, or lack of motivations, or not to decide, letting their behavior hover in a space of ambiguity. Whether or not he was duped, Isaac was no fool. Although he was blind, with his inner eye he observed Jacob's duplicity in both senses of the word: the quality of being double-faced and double-tongued and the quality of being double. "The voice is the voice of Jacob and the hands are Esau's hands" (Gen. 27:22). Isaac thus challenged Jacob with what would become his existential task: to overcome his duplicity by integrating his voice and his hands, his mind and his body.

After Jacob took Esau's birthright and then his blessing, Esau "seethed with resentment" against his brother and vowed to kill him (Gen. 27:41). Helped again by his mother, Jacob fled to her brother Laban in Haran. On the way "he came upon a certain place and stopped there for the night," sleeping on a pillow of stones and dreaming about a ladder (Gen. 28:10–12). It was planted on the ground with its head reaching toward the heavens, and messengers of God were going up and coming down it. Above the ladder stood the LORD, who promised Jacob that the LORD would be with him and would grant him and his seed bountiful increase.

Awestruck, Jacob awakened from his dream and said, "Indeed the LORD is in this place, and I did not know" (Gen. 28:16); in Hebrew, *Acheyn yesh Adonay bamaqom hazeh ve-anochi lo yadati.* The spiritual depth of Jacob's statement can be measured by the multiple interpretations of his utterance. Seven are offered in the book-length meditation by Rabbi Lawrence Kushner titled *God Was in This Place and I, i Did Not Know*: awareness, egotism, the other side, self-reflection, history, the self of the universe, and self.

Several of these interpretations focus on one word in Jacob's utterance, *anochi*, meaning "I." To my ear the word *anochi* is midway between *ani*, meaning "I," and *anachnu*, meaning "we," somewhat analogous to the royal we in English. Like all Hebrew verbs in the past tense, *yadati*, meaning "I knew," contains the subject I as a suffix. Hence the plain sense of Jacob's utterance would be identical if the apparently redundant I of *anochi* were missing. However, according to a cardinal tenet of Biblical interpretation, nothing in the Hebrew Bible is arbitrary or wasted. The presence of an apparent redundancy such as *anochi* in Genesis 28:16 is a signal that something deeper is being implied here.

Rabbi Kushner points out a beautiful interpretation of this extra I by Rabbi Pinchas Horowitz, the author of an important commentary on the Torah. He suggested that it is the direct object of the verb "know," translating the last half of Jacob's statement as "and my I/*anochi* I did not know" or more pointedly as "and my ego-self/*anochi* I did not know." This annulment of the ego-self is what allowed Jacob to perceive God in his dream:

> It is only possible for a person to attain that high rung of being able to say: "Surely God is in this

place," when he or she has utterly eradicated all trace of ego from his or her personality, from his or her sense of self, and from his or her being.

The word *anochi* in Jacob's statement also echoes a word spoken by God during Jacob's dream. "And look, I/*Anochi* am with you and I will guard you wherever you go" (Gen. 28:15). As we noted earlier in this chapter in our discussion of the letter *aleph*, *anochi* is the first word of the Ten Commandments. They begin with the phrase usually translated as "I am the LORD your God," but could also be rendered as "I/*Anochi* is [the name of] the LORD your God." Thus, when Jacob says, "Indeed the LORD is in this place, *ve-anochi lo yadati*," he is also saying, "Indeed the LORD is in this place, and the LORD God I did not know." Thus, rather than referring to his own ego-self as in Rabbi Horowitz's interpretation, in this second reading Jacob is referring to the self of the universe, the oceanic I of primary being of which Jacob's I is a wave. Jacob's relationship with God is our own relationship with God, as Rabbi Rami Shapiro explains in *The Way of Solomon: Finding Joy and Contentment in the Wisdom of Ecclesiastes*:

> We are the waves of the Divine, of the Infinite, of God. We are God in temporary extension. The extent to which we insist on being other, being permanent and separate from each other and God, is the extent to which we are sad, depressed, anxious, lost, and joyless. The extent to which we see the fundamental emptiness of this illusion and awake to the essential unity of all things in, with, and as God is the extent to which we are alive, vibrant, energized, purposeful, and filled with holy joy.

Awakening from the nightmare of duplicity to the essential unity of all things in, with, and as God, Jacob the poet pointed at the stone pillow where he had his dream and punningly proclaimed, *"Acheyn yesh Adonay bamaqom hazeh ve-anochi lo yadati /* Indeed the LORD is in this place, and I did not know" (Gen. 28:16). In so doing, Jacob made a multifaceted wordplay not only on *anochi*, but also on *maqom*, meaning "place."

In the story in chapter 28 of Genesis the word *maqom*/place is repeated six times, signaling, like most repetitions in the Hebrew Bible, the centrality of the concept. It first appears after Jacob escaped from his brother and reached the place where he would have his dream. "And he came upon a certain place — *va-yifga bamaqom* — and stopped there for the night" (Gen. 28:11). In the tradition of the great Rabbinic commentators, we pose a question that focuses on a slight grammatical aberration. Why does the text read *bamaqom*, literally, "upon the place," rather than *bemaqom*, meaning "upon a place"? After all, the place has not yet been identified.

For an answer we refer to Rashi. Concluding that the place must already be known, Rashi identifies it with Mount Moriah, the site of the near-sacrifice of Jacob's father Isaac. "On the third day Abraham raised his eyes and saw *hamaqom*/the place from afar" (Gen. 22:4). Thus in using the word *maqom*/place when he awakened from his dream, Jacob established a connection with the near-sacrifice of his father Isaac, which haunted his family and would haunt the Jewish people throughout history.

Abraham Delson, a student in a Bible class I taught on Jacob's dream, discovered a new interpretation of the phrase *bamaqom hazeh* / in this place. The phrase is self-referential, pointing to itself in this very place in the Hebrew Bible, proclaiming that God is present in the wordplay and multiplicity of interpretation of this very passage. In playing with the text of the Hebrew Bible, Jacob became God's partner. Filled with holy joy over his deepening relationship with God, Jacob exclaimed, "How awe-inspiring is this place!" (translation of Gen. 28:17 by Everett Fox). Jacob had reason to be awestruck. In discovering God in a pile of stones, he discovered his poetic voice.

Jacob's interaction with God while sleeping on the stone pillow was the beginning of his transformation. But his trickery against his father and his brother had conditioned his mind to continue plotting, planning, and conniving. Despite the profundity of the insight when he awoke from his dream — "Indeed the Lord is in this place, and I did not know." — Jacob tainted his transformation by not accepting God unconditionally and wholeheartedly. Instead, he made a deal. The Lord would be his God if the Lord would fulfill the promises He had already made to Jacob in his dream (Gen. 28:20–22). Doubting the veracity of the dream-vision, Jacob remained the heel-grasper, not letting go of a future that he wanted desperately to control.

Despite his lingering blindness to the truth and his refusal to let go, Jacob was energized by his interaction with God, completing the multi-hundred mile journey to Haran, the home of his Uncle Laban, in a single verse, almost in a single stride, as if he were being propelled by Hermes' winged sandals. "And Jacob lifted his feet and went on to the land of the Easterners" (Gen. 29:1).

Jacob labored in Haran for twenty years, acquiring two wives and two concubines, eleven sons and a daughter and extensive wealth. When the Lord told him to return to the land of his fathers, Jacob began the journey home (Gen. 31:3). First he confronted the nameless adversary near the bank of the Yabboq River, at a place he called Peniel, and then he confronted his brother Esau, from whom Jacob had escaped because Esau wanted to kill him.

As Jacob was traveling toward the confrontation with Esau, the text allows us to gaze into Jacob's heart. Heavily laden with oxen and donkeys and sheep, with cattle and camels and male and female slaves, with two wives and two concubines and many children and with a conscience consumed with guilt over how he had double-dealt against his twin brother, "Jacob was greatly afraid, and he was distressed" (Gen. 32:8). Jacob acted out the duplicity that was his hallmark by dividing into two camps the people and the animals that were with him. Then he contrived what seemed to be the perfect plan. Instructing his servants precisely what they should say to Esau, Jacob sent a tribute to his brother, wave after wave of she-goats and he-goats, ewes and rams, cows and bulls, in order to placate him.

Among the most effective artifices used by the Hebrew Bible for portraying the unportrayable encounter with God are the repetition, transformation, and interweaving of keywords such as *anochi*/I and *maqom*/place. As we have seen with both of these examples, a repetition of a keyword in different parts of the text establishes a link among those parts, revealing unexpected connections that otherwise might have been overlooked.

In the text surrounding Jacob's confrontation with Esau, the following keyword cluster is crucial: *panim*, meaning "face," and other words having the same root, such as *lifney*, meaning "ahead of" or "in the face of." The keyword *panim* splinters into sparks in Genesis 32:21–22, where derivatives of this word are repeated five times, each repetition yielding a new meaning. These two verses reveal both Jacob's verbal agility and his obsessiveness as he planned to confront Esau's face (translation by Everett Fox):

"I will wipe (the anger from) his face/*panav* with the gift that goes ahead of my face/*lefanay*; afterward, when I see his face/*panav*, perhaps he will lift up my face/*panay*! The gift crossed over ahead of his face/*panav*. . . ."

Before Jacob would meet Esau, there intervened a night that was to be a night of Jacob's deepening spiritual transformation. The singularity of this night is signaled in the next three verses by another, double wordplay on Jacob's Hebrew name, *Yaaqov/Yabboq/va-ye-aveq*. He brought his family and all his belongings across the *Yabboq* crossing. "And Jacob/*Yaaqov* was left alone, and a man wrestled/*va-ye-aveq* with him until the break of dawn" (Gen. 32:25). We are puzzled by the seeming redundancy of the first half of the verse. It is obvious that after Jacob had stripped himself of family and all other attachments, he was left alone. Why are we told this? Another problem is that the second half of the verse seems to contradict the first half. Although Jacob was left alone, he was not really alone for "a man wrestled with him until the break of dawn."

These apparent inconsistencies invite us to search for another reading. The first half of Genesis 32:25, "And Jacob was left alone," is a translation of the Hebrew, *va-yivater Yaaqov levado*. Changing the vowels in the first of the three words yields *ve-yoter*, which is Hebrew for "and more." Thus the phrase, "And Jacob was left alone," can also be read as "And alone Jacob was more" or "And alone Jacob became more." With this interpretation Genesis 32:25 highlights Jacob's deepening transformation as a Zen koan: Jacob had more by having less. At this moment, the quietest in the chapter, Jacob confronted the unknown adversary as the wrestling match began.

What happened in the interval between Jacob's being alone and the wrestling match goes beyond words. Alone Jacob became more, and a man wrestled with him until the break of dawn. The text tantalizes us by the silence between the two phrases. How did Jacob, the double-dealing, double-faced, double-tongued conniver and heel-sneak, focus his inner resources first upon the struggle with the unknown adversary and then upon the struggle with Esau? Just before this scene, Jacob was obsessively manipulating and controlling, trying to placate his brother with the perfect words and the perfect tribute. But after he had stripped himself of family and all other attachments, Jacob's mind became peaceful. No plans, no artifice, no fear, no words. Just silence.

Alone, Jacob sat on the bank of the Yabboq crossing and meditated. On that dark night, he discovered a new way of being, based not on double-dealing, grasping, and control, but on insight and love.

In so doing, Jacob drew on the legacy of his father, Isaac, who meditated in the field toward evening (Gen. 24:63) and gave his son the gifts of silence and inwardness. In his book on Jewish meditation, Rabbi Alan Lew interprets the ladder and the messengers of God that appeared in Jacob's dream after he had escaped from Esau (Gen. 28:12) as metaphors for meditation. The "image of the ladder," planted on the ground with its head reaching toward the heavens, "is a picture of the human condition in general, but more specifically it is a picture of a human being in meditation." In addition, the messengers of God "going up and down [the ladder] between heaven and earth" are what "we become more conscious of during meditation. But most of all there is the breath, the ultimate, the most decisive divine message — and the most conspicuous object of our awareness during meditation as well."

Alone Jacob became more, and a man wrestled with him until the break of dawn. After the man had wounded Jacob's hip (Gen. 32:26), the opponents began to wrestle with words. The man asked Jacob to let him go, but Jacob refused until the man would bless him, but the man withheld the blessing, asking Jacob for his name, which the man replaced with Israel, in Hebrew *Yisrael*, meaning "God-Fighter" (translation of Gen. 32:29 by Everett Fox). The new name, *Yisrael*, is based on *sarah* or "strive" and *el* or "God." In his book, *God Is a Verb: Kaballah and the Practice of Mystical Judaism,* Rabbi David A. Cooper offers another, beautiful reading that reflects back on Jacob's earlier career. Changing the vowels in *Yisrael* yields *Yashar-el*, meaning "God is straight" or "that which yearns to go directly to God." In his double dealing with Esau twenty years earlier, Esau had punned on Jacob's name to characterize him as a person who acted crookedly. *Yaaqov*, the heel-grasper; *Yaaqov*, the heel-sneak. Now, in preparation for the reunion with his brother, Jacob was wounded and then healed, made straight by the model of God.

The impossibility of identifying the adversary shrouds the wrestling match in mystery. Where did he come from? Was it another dream? As Robert Alter emphasizes, whether the adversary was an angel, a malignant spirit, or the personification of Jacob's fear, the psychological component is clear:

> Appearing to Jacob in the dark of the night, before the morning when Esau will be reconciled with Jacob, he is the embodiment of portentous antagonism in Jacob's dark night of the soul. He is obviously in some sense a doubling of Esau as adversary, but he is also a doubling of all with which Jacob has had to contend. . . .

Alone Jacob became more by facing his double nature in the person of the adversary, the "externalization of all that Jacob has to wrestle with within himself."

A revealing exchange with the nameless adversary occurred after Jacob had won his new name. And Jacob asked and said, "Tell your name, pray" (Gen. 32:30). Jacob has just meditated. Memories of his former existence bubbled up from his subconscious: the conniving, the double-dealing, the verbal gymnastics. Doubt was arising, and the urge to hold onto the wrestling match by giving his adversary a name, and the urge to construct a story around the memories, congealing them into a solid, substantial reality.

Having canceled the curse of Jacob's birth name, *Yaaqov*, by replacing it with *Yisrael*, the nameless adversary would next help Jacob transcend the limitations of all names. The man's reply, "Why should you ask my name?", jolted Jacob into understanding. Names — *Yaaqov*, the heel-grasper; *Yaaqov*, the heel-sneak; *Yisrael*, God-Fighter — are concepts that freeze experience, violating the universal law of impermanence and change. Constructing a story around the memories and naming them would bring more suffering. I am *Yaaqov*, who craved and won Esau's birthright and Esau's blessing. I am *Yisrael*, who has "striven with God and men, and won out" (Gen. 32:29). Only by letting go of the past, only by letting the nameless adversary and all of experience remain nameless could the former heel-grasper face his brother. Jacob's awakening to the addictive power of all names and all concepts was the true blessing of his night of transformation.*
The man saw in Jacob's face that he understood, "and there he blessed him" (Gen. 32:30).

---

* This interpretation of Genesis 32:30 was inspired by Rhonda Shapiro-Rieser. Several of the insights in this paragraph are due to her.

Spiritual growth is slow, and old addictions linger. Immediately, Jacob violated the adversary's lesson by naming the place of his awakening. "And Jacob called the name of the place Peniel, meaning, 'I have seen God face to face / *panim el panim* and I came out alive'" (Gen. 32:31). Then Jacob remembered what he had just learned. Having just given the name Peniel to the place of his awakening, in the very next verse he changed it. "And the sun rose upon him as he passed Penuel and he was limping on his hip" (Gen. 32:32). Jacob, the poet who had discovered the silence beyond words, changed Peniel into Penuel. In freezing experience, names create the illusion of a solid, substantial reality; buying into that reality causes suffering. But Jacob had suffered enough. He had caused himself to suffer. He had caused others to suffer. The past was over.

"And the sun rose upon him as he passed Penuel and he was limping on his hip." The sun shined upon Jacob the calm light of insight and awareness, the fruits of Jacob's twenty years in exile and his night of struggle with the nameless adversary. The pain from his wounded hip was the unavoidable pain of being alive and gaining insight. The wounded hip is never mentioned again because, as Jacob understood, pain is inevitable, but suffering, *dukkha*, is not.

"And Jacob called the name of the place Peniel, meaning, 'I have seen God face to face / *panim el panim* and I came out alive'" (Gen. 32:31). Obsessed until the struggle at Peniel with double-dealing, grasping, and control, Jacob confronted the nameless adversary and himself face to face / *panim el panim*. Transcending his duplicity, Jacob, the wordsmith become wrestler, integrated in this struggle the hands of Esau and his own voice (Gen. 27:22). He was then ready for the face-to-face encounter with his brother, which he would execute skillfully and elegantly.

Transformed by his insight into impermanence and change, Jacob mindfully faced his next challenge. He "raised his eyes and saw and, look, Esau was coming, and with him were four hundred men" (Gen. 33:1). Without artifice, fear, or words, Jacob accepted whatever would happen with perfect trust. "And he . . . bowed to the ground seven times until he drew near his brother. And Esau ran to meet him and embraced him and fell upon his neck and kissed him, and they wept" (Gen. 33:3–4). Like Jacob, the reader is astonished by Esau's actions. As Avivah Gottlieb Zornberg points out in her study of the Book of Genesis, Esau's physicality reminds us of the wrestling match with the nameless adversary. Jacob introduced his family to Esau and then addressed him using the same keyword *panim*/face that he used in the naming ceremony at Peniel, meaning "Face of God." "O, no, pray, if I have found favor in your eyes, take this tribute from my hand," begs the contrite younger brother, "for have I not seen your face/*panecha* as one might see God's face / *pney Elohim*, and you received me in kindness?" (Gen. 33:10).

Finally, mercifully, Jacob was at peace, a state of mind made possible by Esau's equally-astonishing transformation. Esau forgave his younger brother, who had wounded him so deeply. Esau forgave him because Esau saw Jacob's contrition in his face. It was Jacob's face, not the lavish gifts and not the honeyed words, that brought him reconciliation and peace. Filled with guilt, desiring atonement, and ultimately forgiven, Jacob revealed to Esau the hidden blessing of his heart: "God has favored me and I have everything" (Gen. 33:11). "And Jacob came in peace to the town of Shechem, which is in the land of Canaan" (Gen. 33:18). In peace, *shalem*, finally whole.

Jacob's story is a story of transformation: how a person focused on achievement and control discovers, through suffering, struggle, and meditation, a new way of being, based on insight and love; how a person who craved to construct a story around the difficult experiences of his past, congealing them into a solid, substantial reality and then suffering from that solidification, learned to let go. Jacob's story touches me deeply because his transformation is my own. Jacob's face brought him peace. My face brought me peace.

Jacob's story of transformation continues to unfold for another 17 chapters, until the end of Genesis. Its energy radiates through the Hebrew Bible both via the power of his awakening and via keywords such as *panim*/face, which set up links with other key passages in the Hebrew Bible. Creation in Genesis 1:2: "when the earth was wild and waste, darkness over the face of Ocean, rushing-spirit of God hovering over the face of the waters / *al pney hamayim*" (translation by Everett Fox). The dreadful infinitude of God's face in Exodus 33:20: "And He said, 'You shall not be able to see My face/*panay*, for no human can see Me and live.'" The healing infinitude of God's face in the priestly blessing (Numbers 6:24–26):

> May the LORD bless you and guard you.
> May the LORD shine His face/*panav* to you and grant grace to you.
> May the LORD lift up His face/*panav* to you and give you peace.

And may the LORD lift up His face/*panav* to you, the reader. May the LORD give you peace by opening up to you what Jacob learned about pain and suffering and the peace that comes from letting go.

Like Jacob, we have traveled a great distance in this chapter, starting with the basic paradox at the heart of the Hebrew Bible's narrative art. How can words express the encounter between humans and God, who is beyond all words? As the examples in this chapter and the next two chapters suggest, the Hebrew language of the Bible is different from other human discourse. Written without vowels or punctuation and based on three-letter consonantal roots, it is an ideal medium to describe the intensity and depth of the human-Divine encounter, doing so through literary artifices such as paradox, wordplay, puns, and ambiguity, which flow naturally from the structure of the language itself.

Particularly in some of its narrative portions, the ambiguity of the Hebrew Bible is so pervasive and the text is so open-ended that the reader's participation becomes necessary. Rabbi Louis Finkelstein describes how these features of the text are fundamental to Rabbinic thought:

> That the text is at once perfect and perpetually incomplete; that like the universe itself it was created to be a process rather than a system — a method of inquiry into the right, rather than a codified collection of answers; that to discover possible situations with which it might deal and to analyze their moral implications in the light of its teachings is to share the labour of Divinity — these are inherent elements of Rabbinic thought, dominating the manner of life it recommends.

The perfect, yet perpetually and intentionally incomplete text of the Hebrew Bible beams a message to us. Play with me, it urges. Wrestle with me, as Jacob did with the unknown adversary at Peniel. Continue to splinter me into sparks of new meanings by interpreting and reinterpreting me. In so doing, you will face, and will be blessed by, the multilayered ambiguity and interconnectedness and open-endedness of your own life. In the same way that you read the Hebrew Bible, so will you live.

Sensitized by the Jacob narrative to the indeterminacy, ambiguity, interconnectedness, and open-endedness of the text and of our lives, we will next read the story of creation in chapter 1 of Genesis and the Garden of Eden story in chapters 2 and 3.

5
Conceptual Thinking Banishes Us from Eden

> [B]efore the creation, the Torah was nothing more than a heap of letters which could have been arranged in any order. When Adam sinned, they rose and arranged themselves in the order we know today. When the Messiah comes, they will unravel themselves like knitting and create a new Torah, a new heaven and a new earth.
> — Tamar Yellin, *The Genizah at the House of Shepher*

IN THE LAST CHAPTER we read the narrative of Jacob, which in the original Hebrew is energized by a dynamic wordplay. The unpredictability and creativity of the transformations of Jacob's name mirror the potential for creative change in Jacob's character, each transformation corresponding to a crucial episode in his life. During the wrestling match, the unknown adversary conveyed to Jacob a basic Buddhist teaching about the limitations of all names. Names are concepts that freeze experience and so violate the universal law of impermanence and change. For Jacob, letting go of names was letting go of the past, in which he cheated both his brother and his father. The epitome of the clever Jew who had prevailed by his wit and his guile, Jacob discovered a new way of being, based not on achievement and control, but on insight and love.

A dynamic wordplay resonating deeply with Buddhist teachings on the genesis of self-consciousness, the birth of the ego-self, and the possibility of enlightenment also energizes the two narratives that we will now examine, the story of creation and the story of the Garden of Eden in chapters 1, 2, and 3 of Genesis. In translation, these narratives have become widely used conceptual lenses for interpreting many of our experiences involving creativity, gender, sex, sin, banishment, relationship with God, relationship with self, and more. In this chapter we examine other faces of these root narratives by turning their conceptual lenses back on themselves. In doing this, we will see that the story of creation and the story of the Garden of Eden also elucidate a basic Buddhist theme: the genesis of conceptual thinking and how one may go beyond it.

Without conceptual thinking, the finite human mind cannot interpret the infinite complexity of reality. We need concepts of time such as past, present, future, youth, and old age. Concepts of ownership: this is my body, my mind, my pain. Concepts of gender, nationality, race, money, spirituality, God, Buddha nature, and enlightenment. However, concepts create duality: I and you, good and bad, pleasure and pain. Concepts create separation: I versus you, good versus bad, pleasure versus pain. Concepts create boundaries. We invest concepts with a magical power that leads to suffering when we define each term as the negation, and eventually the exclusion, of its opposite in what seems to be an inevitable process of conceptualization, dualization, and separation.

As David Loy points out in his book, *Money, Sex, War, Karma: Notes for a Buddhist Revolution,* this process is explained by a fundamental Buddhist teaching. Although we think that we are experiencing reality, the world we face through the fog of concepts is an illusion created by the language in which we formulate those concepts:

> [O]ur commonsense view of the world is not commonsense at all, because an unconscious philosophy is actually built into the ways we ordinarily use language. . . . With language as our lens, we perceive the world as a collection of separate things that interact with each other in objective space and time. We separate things from each other by labeling them — that is, by giving them names.

Trying to grasp reality through concepts rather than through direct experience, we suffer, as I did when I cursed and raged against the headache pain, solidifying the concept of pain into the only lens for interpreting my moment-to-moment experience. Thus conditioned, my mind made the inevitable choice, which in turn locked it into a never-ending cycle of aversion and clinging. What increases the pain is bad and is to be avoided. What decreases the pain is good and is to be clung to. And I suffered even more.

In investing concepts with a magical power, we seem to be following God's lead during the seven days of creation. God's words and actions in the opening verses of Genesis seem to focus upon creating duality, separation, and boundaries:

> [A]nd God divided the light from the darkness. And God called the light Day, and the darkness He called Night. (Gen. 1:4–5)
>
> And God said, "Let there be a vault in the midst of the waters, and let it divide the water from water." . . . [A]nd so it was. (Gen. 1:6–7)
>
> And God said, "Let the waters under the heavens be gathered in one place so that dry land will appear," and so it was. (Gen. 1:9)
>
> And God said, "Let there be lights in the vault of the heavens to divide the day from the night. . . ." And so it was. (Gen. 1:14–15)

Light and darkness, day and night, the waters beneath divided from the waters above by the vault of the heavens, dry land and seas, the sun and the moon. From the perspective of the finite human mind interacting with the infinite Divine mind, God conceptualizes creation.

In doing this, God foreshadows the genesis of the most seductive concept of all, which is born in the Garden of Eden: the concept of the ego-self, the root concept in which we invest our energy, feeding it, protecting it, using it to create and then to solidify the boundary cutting ourselves off from the world and the source of all being.

Eve and Adam ate the fruit of the tree of knowledge of good and evil, concerning which God had commanded Adam not to eat (Gen 2:17). Sexual awakening. Self-consciousness was born, as was the awareness of duality and separation. "And the eyes of the two were opened, and they knew they were naked, and they sewed fig leaves and made themselves loincloths" (Gen. 3:7). God then asked Adam, "Where are you?" (Gen. 3:9). Adam responded, "I heard Your sound in the garden and I was afraid, for I was naked, and I hid" (Gen. 3:10). Adam spoke about himself, the momentous first act of self-reference by a human in the Hebrew Bible. Consciousness doubles back on itself to discover an independent, agitated, and fearful ego-self. "I was afraid, for I was naked, and I hid."

We are Eve and Adam. Their story is the drama of our being born, maturing, suffering, and awakening. According to the text, God punished Eve and Adam and drove them out of the garden. Developmentally, however, the punishment and the banishment are self-imposed. We are born whole. As it is the nature of the trees in the garden to beget fruit, so it is the nature of our minds to beget self-consciousness. Concepts separate us from reality and from our Buddha nature as we drive ourselves out of the garden of childhood innocence. Fraught with anxiety, we spend a lifetime trying to reenter. But concepts cannot be canceled by yet more concepts.

A new way of being, unmediated by any conceptual lens, is required. The teachings of the Buddha and the wisdom of the Hebrew Bible show us the way. Especially in the early chapters of Genesis, the Hebrew Bible speaks a Buddhist language that goes beyond words by not investing them with fixed meanings, but by recognizing that they are empty, a Buddhist concept conveying not a meaningless void, but a dynamic, interconnected web of significance devoid of any defining essence and therefore pregnant with possibility.

As we experience the story of Eve and Adam in the garden, we confront the drama of our own suffering, which is summarized in the Buddha's Four Noble Truths: the truth of the existence of suffering, the truth of the origin of suffering, the truth of the end of suffering, the way leading to the end of suffering. How will the Four Noble Truths manifest themselves in our own lives? How will we discover a new way of being, unmediated by any conceptual lens?

Enlightenment is possible because in themselves concepts are not the problem. They are useful mental constructs that divide, chop, and split reality into small compartments that may be analyzed and so understood. The problem arises when we forget that concepts are only mental constructs and we allow them to violate the Buddha's basic insights about the nature of reality. Reality is impermanent, spontaneously flowing and changing on every level. Devoid of any defining essence, reality is a dynamic, interconnected web of significance pregnant with possibility.

The Buddha exposed the truly radical nature of these insights when he formulated his most distinctive and counter-intuitive teaching, which totally contradicts the conventional understanding of society. This is the teaching that there is no fixed self at the core of our experiences, a teaching made accessible and experientially obvious through meditation. Just as reality is impermanent, spontaneously flowing and changing on every level, so is the self impermanent. Joseph Goldstein, a co-founder of the Insight Meditation Society, has been leading meditation retreats worldwide since 1974. In his Dharma talk on concepts and reality, he analogizes the illusion of a fixed self to the illusion of the Big Dipper in the night sky:

> There is no Big Dipper. There are some points of lights which we call stars, and . . . we have separated out one particular group of points of light, and we have put a concept on it: Big Dipper. . . . When you have become so conditioned to see patterns in a certain way, to have these concepts

so strong in our minds, it is very difficult to simplify our perception to see just what there is. In exactly the same way that the Big Dipper is a concept, the idea of a self, the idea of "I" is also a concept. What we are is a constellation of changing elements of mind and body, and then we put this idea of self on it.

When we do not understand the nature of reality and the impermanence of self, we live in illusion and the appearance of things and we suffer. Forgetting that concepts are merely mental constructs, we allow them to freeze the flow, stop the change, mechanize the spontaneity, and condition the mind with the illusion that we can control the show. Until we understand the nature of this conditioning, concepts delude us. This delusion, in turn, brings suffering in the Buddhist sense of *dukkha*, the pervasive uncertainty and stress and anxiety arising from the sense that things are not quite right, that I constantly have to be doing rather than just be, that the wheel will stop turning after I publish another paper or earn more praise or earn more money. But the next paper and the next piece of praise and the next chunk of money make the wheel turn even faster.

Reading the narratives of creation and the Garden of Eden in the original Hebrew reveals insights that resonate deeply with Buddhist teachings on conceptual thinking and the birth of the ego-self and that elucidate them. These insights are unavailable in translation, where they are often obscured beneath a veneer of conventional interpretation. The Garden of Eden story, we will see, is infinitely more than just a story about sin. When we read the text with a sensitivity to the original Hebrew, we will be invited not to solidify concepts by defining them as the negation and eventually the exclusion of their opposites. In the original language, the Hebrew Bible Buddhistly invites us to regard these conceptual pairs as dynamic word-clusters involving interdependent processes.

This approach to reading the Hebrew Bible is consistent with a basic insight that meditation has taught me concerning the incoherence of the headaches. I have often experienced days of total relaxation and nights of sound sleep, followed by mornings when I feel the pain churning in my nose. I meditate. Sometimes the pain disappears, and sometimes it worsens. I have also experienced days of stress and agitation followed by nights of fractured sleep. Yet when I wake up, I am pain-free. I meditate, and sometimes I remain pain-free, and sometimes the pain coagulates out of thought and breath and flows tempestuously into my nose, and sometimes it dissipates. The pain has a life of its own, which I can't control and can't understand. The Buddha called this insight *anatta* or selflessness. Bodily processes cannot be governed, nor do they happen according to our wishes.

The Hebrew Bible mirrors the incoherence of bodily processes by giving us incoherent narratives, which invite us to search deeper. When Adam disobeyed God's commandment not to eat the fruit of the tree of knowledge of good and evil, God punished Eve with pain in childbirth and subservience to her husband. How could God expect humans to be honest when God wasn't honest? God couldn't have issued the commandment to Eve for the simple reason that at the time of the commandment Eve didn't exist. So why did God punish her? That bumper sticker was right: Eve was framed. An important lesson is revealed by this incoherence in the holy text, which traces the genesis of the concept of ego-self only in Adam, not in Eve. Although God punished Eve, she remained whole, and her wholeness could be the seed of future enlightenment that is planted in us and that we must nurture if it is eventually to blossom.

This and other inconsistencies in the Garden of Eden narrative invite us to read it much more closely. First we will examine the story of creation, which it mirrors, distorts, reconfigures, and reinterprets thematically and linguistically. Although the English translation obscures the complexity of the issues, the Hebrew original trumpets the complexity from the very first word.

We start with the symphonic opening of the Book of Genesis as orchestrated by the committee that gave the world the King James translation:

> In the beginning God created the heaven and the earth. And the earth was without form, and void; and darkness was upon the face of the deep. And the Spirit of God moved upon the face of the waters. And God said, Let there be light: and there was light.

The eloquent majesty of these words, coupled with their complete familiarity, might lull us into thinking that the process of creation as recorded in Genesis and, by extrapolation, creation itself were linear and orderly. Not so, as the Hebrew original makes evident. A mystery pervades creation, a mystery that we are excluded from understanding because it includes ourselves.

The mystery of creation is manifested in part in its fractal nature. The term "fractal" was coined by the mathematician Benoit B. Mandelbrot, who defines it as "a set for which the Hausdorff-Besicovitch dimension strictly exceeds the topological dimension." Like a packed poetic line that evokes a world after it is deciphered, for those who have been initiated into the mysteries of mathematics Mandelbrot's definition is a seed that generates the bountiful tree of fractal geometry, which his text and many others explore. However, to the non-mathematician the concept of a fractal remains opaque and impenetrable, like the Hebrew Bible to those who do not understand Hebrew.

In the present book fractal is used in a poetic sense to refer to objects having properties analogous to those of mathematical fractals. Scale invariance and self-similarity are the buzzwords. In general, an object has fractal-like properties if it exhibits a similar form on smaller and smaller scales, each small portion of the whole a replica of the whole. In this extended sense it describes many fragmented and irregular shapes appearing in nature. Their hallmark is that the degree of their fragmentation and irregularity is similar at all scales.

Mathematical examples of fractals abound. One can also see fractals in nature as in a fern, a seacoast, or a branching tree. Whether one looks at these shapes from far away or up close, one sees the same pattern. Consider a tree trunk splitting into boughs, then branches, then limbs and twigs and stems of increasingly smaller size. The branchings of a twig on one of these limbs, branching into every smaller twiglets and stems, has a similar shape as the whole.

The objects included in the poetic universe of fractals go beyond mathematics to include not only objects in nature such as a fern or a seacoast or a branching tree, but also the Torah and the first word of the Torah, *bereyshit*, usually translated as "in the beginning" but having a mystical depth inaccessible in any translation.

The essence of a fractal is that the shape of the whole is mirrored in the shape of portions of the whole. Thus in a fractal the whole can be reproduced from such portions. This is the fractal essence of life itself. The complexity of the universe is replicated in the complexity of each life-form, which contains the seed that reproduces the next generation of itself from a portion of itself. The Torah reveals this truth in the record of the third day of creation when the first life-form is created (Gen. 1:11–12):

> And God said, "Let the earth grow grass, plants yielding seed of each kind and trees bearing fruit of each kind, that has its seed within it upon the earth." And so it was.

The Zohar, the primary text of Jewish mysticism, also contains a potent fractal-insight. According to the Zohar, the fractal structure of the universe is reflected in the Torah, and, as the following quotation shows, the fractal structure of the Torah is in turn reflected in the Decalogue or Ten Commandments. In this quotation the term "Ten Words" is used to refer both to the Ten Commandments and to God's ten creative utterances during creation, of which the first was "Let there be light" in Genesis 1:3:

> Rabbi Eleazar taught that in the Ten Words [Decalogue] all the other commandments were engraved, with all decrees and punishments, all laws concerning purity and impurity, all the branches and roots, all the trees and plants, heaven and earth, seas and oceans, in fact, all things. For the Torah is the Name of the Holy One of Being. As the Name of the Holy One is engraved in the Ten Words [creative utterances] of Creation, so is the whole Torah engraved in the Ten Words

[Decalogue], and these Ten Words are the Name
of the Holy One, and the whole Torah is thus
one Name, the Holy Name of God.

The mystery of creation, both fractal and otherwise, is also expressed by the first word of the Hebrew original of Genesis, *bereyshit*, which is the Hebrew name of the first book of the Bible. *Bereyshit* is the first word of a sentence that most people are surprised to learn was mistranslated by the King James committee and also seems to contain a grammatical error in the original Hebrew.

We will soon explore the complex, fractal nature of *bereyshit*. Its complexity mirrors the profundity of the sentence of which it is the first word, a sentence pregnant with ambiguity, mystery, and multiple meaning.* The grammatical form of the first word *bereyshit* causes Rashi to reject the reading "In the beginning God created the heaven and the earth," which was used in the King James Bible. In his opinion the plain sense of the verse is the following: "In the beginning of God's creation of the heaven and the earth" or "When God created the heaven and the earth." Rather than the beginning of time as suggested by the King James translation, Rashi's reading calls our attention to the beginning of a process that, as in Buddhist belief, could be recurring. His understanding is that the first two verses of Genesis set the stage for the creation of light in the third verse.

Rashi gives another reason for this alternate reading besides syntax. The translation, "In the beginning God created the heaven

---

* This discussion summarizes insights of the great Torah sages, Rashi and Ramban (also called Nachmanides). They are taken from two translations of Rashi's commentary on Genesis by Rabbi Avrohom Davis and Rabbi Meir Zlotowitz and from the translation of Ramban's commentary on Genesis by Rabbi Dr. Charles B. Chavel.

and the earth," suggests that the Torah is giving the chronological order of the acts of creation. But this interpretation is contradicted by Genesis 1:2, which tells of "God's breath hovering over the waters." According to Rashi, Genesis 1:2 proves that the waters must have preceded the creation of the heaven and the earth in Genesis 1:1. However, the Torah does not indicate when the waters were created.

An inconsistency between the first two words of Genesis 1:1 energizes Rashi's commentary. His reading of this verse as "In the beginning of God's creation of the heaven and the earth" is inconsistent with the traditional, vocalized form of the second word, translated here as "creation." The vowels in this word must be changed if Rashi's reading is to make sense. In order to resolve the inconsistency, Rashi prefers a metaphorical interpretation that depends on another meaning of the first word *bereyshit*.

The word *bereyshit* consists of the common and ambiguous preposition *be*, which has the various senses of "in," "with," "for," or "for the sake of," and the noun *reyshit*, meaning "the beginning of." In order to interpret the opening verse of Genesis, Rashi cites Jeremiah 2:3 and Proverbs 8:22, which single out two entities of great significance that are called *reyshit*: the Torah and Israel. This leads to another reading of Genesis 1:1: "For the sake of (*be*) [the Torah and Israel which bear the name of] *reyshit*, God created the heaven and the earth."

"For the sake of the Torah, God created the heaven and the earth." This interpretation of the first verse of the Torah confers an infinite significance on that text. From here it is a small step to the Rabbinic teaching that in fact the Torah was the blueprint of creation preceding creation. Only after the Torah was consulted could God's creation begin. According to one commentary

(*Bereyshit Rabbah* 1:1), "The Holy One, blessed be He, . . . looked into the Torah and created the world."

Conceptualizing the Torah as the blueprint of creation has profound textual implications. As Susan Handelman points out in her book, *The Slayers of Moses: The Emergence of Rabbinic Interpretation in Modern Literary Theory*, these implications can be realized through the act of interpretation:

> [W]ith the proper methods of interpretation, one can unlock the mysteries of all being. Every crownlet of every letter is filled with significance, and even the forms of letters are hints to profound meaning. To understand creation, one looks not to nature but to the Torah; the world can be read out of the Torah, and the Torah read from the world.

Through the act of interpretation, we again confront the fractal nature of reality. The Torah is part of the world, which in turn can be read out of the Torah.

Because the text lacks vowels and punctuation, because of multiple ambiguities at the levels of letters, words, and verses, meaning in the Torah is not an absolute quality of the text alone. Rather, meaning is the fruit of the reader's interaction with the text. As a result of this interaction, the human relationship with God and the personality of God portrayed in the text do not remain static. The reader's perceptions of her relationship with God and of God's personality change as the reader's experiences change.

Besides these readings, the first verse of Genesis can be read in numerous other ways. Several of these focus on the root of *bereyshit*, which is *rosh*, meaning "head." The root meaning becomes apparent if one moves the last two letters of *bereyshit* to the next word and inserts different vowels, obtaining a word meaning "will create himself." This movement of letters is not unreasonable since in ancient Torah scrolls not only were vowels and punctuation missing, but also the spaces between individual words. With these alterations, Genesis 1:1 can also be read as follows: "In his head God will create himself [along] with the heaven and the earth." This interpretation is consistent with mystical insights that the universe is a thought in God's mind.

As we read the opening verse of the Torah, our interaction with the text releases a cornucopia of different interpretations: "In the beginning of God's creation"; "For the sake of the Torah God created"; "In his head God will create." All these readings are inexhaustibly enriched by their interactions with the thousands of verses that follow, an infinite orchard of interpretation that blossoms from the astonishingly fertile first word *bereyshit*.

"In the beginning God created the heaven and the earth." This is the majestic opening verse of the King James Bible, which reproduces word for word the translation in Jerome's Vulgate. In the King James Bible, this opening verse introduces a lucid narrative of the logical, orderly creation of the universe. However, reading the Hebrew text through the lenses of Rashi's commentary and those of others is a totally different experience. Through these lenses the unfathomable and open-ended mystery of creation becomes apparent. "There is a tension," Avivah Gottlieb Zornberg writes, "between the benevolent clarity and power of the narrative and the acknowledgment of mystery that inheres in the very first word and that develops as the implications of the beginning are realized."

Bereyshit, the first word of the Hebrew original of Genesis and the Hebrew name of the book as a whole, expresses the fractal nature of creation in an extraordinary symbiosis of form and meaning on multiple levels. The first two letters of *bereyshit* are *bet* and *resh*. The first letter *bet*, in its printed form ב, contains inside itself the second letter *resh*, printed as ר. The letters *bet* and *resh* are also respective forms of the Hebrew words *bayit* and *rosh*, meaning "house" and "head." What occurs on the level of letters, the *resh* inside the *bet*, mirrors what occurs on the level of words. Namely, the six-letter word *bereyshit* consists of the word *rosh* (letters 2, 3, 4) literally inside the word *bayit* (letters 1, 5, 6).* And what occurs on the level of words mirrors what occurs on the level of the verse, connecting back to the main narrative and significantly deepening our understanding of it. Namely, mystical commentary on the Torah regards the *rosh*/head inside the *bayit*/house in the six-letter word *bereyshit* as signifying the male sex organ inside the female sex organ engaged in the act of sexual intercourse that engendered the universe. This reading, in turn, connects human sexuality with divine sexuality, conferring great significance upon the former and foreshadowing one of the main themes of the dream narrative that unfolds in the Garden of Eden. The woman and the man eat the fruit from the tree of knowledge of good and evil and discover their sexuality.

That *bereyshit* works on all three levels of letters, words, and verse, each mirroring the other, reveals the fractal structure of *bereyshit*. Its complexity mirrors the fractal structure of the Torah, of which it is the first word. In addition, since God looked into the Torah before creating the world, *bereyshit* also expresses the fractal structure of the universe, the creation of which begins with *bereyshit*.

---

* In Hebrew *bereyshit* is בראשית, in which *rosh*/ראש (letters 2, 3, 4) is inside *bayit*/בית (letters 1, 5, 6).

After sampling these many insights into *bereyshit*, it should come as no surprise that mystical thought venerates that potent cluster of six Hebrew letters in verse 1 of the Torah as the Big Bang of creation, into which the infinite energy of the Torah is compacted. In their book, *Letters to a Buddhist Jew*, Akiva Tatz and David Gottlieb explain the generative power of *bereyshit*:

> One begins with Genesis, the moment of firstness in which all is coded. Torah sources make clear that the entire Torah can be derived from the first word "Bereishit [sic] — In the beginning. . .;" its manifold permutations indicate all that is to come.

As the second letter of the Hebrew alphabet having the numerical value of two, the *bet* with which the word *bereyshit* and the Torah begin has another key function. The letter *bet* summarizes the duality principle that is the main structural feature of Genesis, from the birth of conceptual thinking in the dual creation narratives and the Garden of Eden story to its maturation in the lives of the forefathers, Abraham, Isaac, and Jacob.*

This duality principle is active in the very first verse of the Torah, the first two words of which are *bereyshit* and *bara* ("created"). Not only does *bara* echo the first two syllables of *bereyshit*, but also these two syllables have the same consonants as *bara*, differing only in the vowels. The Hebrew words translated as "God" and as "heaven" also express the duality of creation because both have a plural form, *Elohim* and *shamayim*. When the plural form *Elohim*, meaning "God," is paired with the singular form of the verb *bara*, translated in the King James version as "created,"

---

* This discussion of the duality principle is based in part on the article by Israel Koren and the book by Friedrich Weinreb listed in the Bibliography.

one is reminded that creation was not the smooth process that the King James version suggests.

The duality principle evident in the first verse is reflected in the contents of the days of creation, each of which is based on a sequence of pairs. On the first day, for example, we have heaven and earth (Gen. 1:1), welter and waste (Gen. 1:2), God's breath hovering over the waters (Gen. 1:2), and day and night (Gen. 1:4–5); on the second day we have the water beneath the vault of the heavens and the water above the vault (Gen. 1:6). The duality principle expressed in the first letter and in the first verse and in the contents of the days of creation is also expressed in the division of the six days of creation into two groups of three days each. The first and fourth days both deal with light, the second and fifth days with water, and the third and sixth days with land and the life-forms that God creates upon it.

The dualistic pattern of creation repeats itself in the lives of the forefathers. Abraham is associated with the light, fire, and heat of the first and fourth days of creation: the smoking brazier with a flaming torch (Gen. 15:18), the heat of the day (Gen. 18:1), the destruction of Sodom and Gomorrah through brimstone and fire (Gen. 19:24), and the offering up of his son as a burnt offering (Gen. 22:2).

Isaac, the almost-sacrificed son, is associated with water, which corresponds to the second and fifth days. His wife Rebecca was first seen near a well (Gen. 24:15–20), and Isaac quarreled with Abimelech over the waters of the wells of Gerar (Gen. 26:15–32).

Jacob, the synthesis of Abraham and Isaac, is associated with the life-forms of the third and sixth days of creation: plants, such as the lentils of the stew with which Jacob purchased Esau's birthright (Gen. 25:29–34); animals, such as the livestock he raised while working for Laban (Gen. 30:25–43) and the animals he gave to Esau as a present (Gen. 32:14–20, 33:8–11); and people, particularly his twelve sons, who settled in Egypt and became the progenitors of the nation of Israel, liberated from Egypt during the first Passover.

We come back full circle to the duality of creation because duality also defines Jacob: he had a twin brother Esau; two names, Jacob and Israel; two wives, Rachel and Leah; and two servants, Bilhah and Zilpah. His code word is duplicity in both senses of the word: the quality of double-dealing and the quality of being double.

The duality principle that structures Genesis and is mirrored fractally in Jacob's life also underlies the creation of male and female, which is narrated twice, first in chapter 1 and then in chapter 2. The first creation in chapter 1 is a purely literary one, creating out of pure words a disembodied hermaphrodite, the pure idea of male and female whose only connection to nature is to control it. Here is Genesis 1:26–27 with singular and plural forms of pronouns emphasized; the pronoun "He" in the second and third lines of verse 27 does not appear in the original Hebrew but is indicated by the form of the verb "created." In both verses the Hebrew word translated as "God" is *Elohim*, a plural form coupled with the singular verbs "said" and "created" as in Genesis 1:1. Is the text sloppy in its use of plural forms of pronouns or is it conveying something profound?

> 26: And God said, "Let *us* make a human in our image, by *our* likeness, to hold sway over the fish of the sea. . . .
> 27: And God created the human in *his* image, in the image of God [*He*] created *him*, male and female [*He*] created *them*.

Mirroring the creation of the human in God's image, the last three lines envelop the human with God and God with the human. Male and female, created in God's image, are also dual facets of God: God as *Elohim*, powerful and transcendent, and God as *Shechinah*, conveying God's Mothering Presence, intimate and compassionate (translation by Chaim Stern). In Hebrew "compassion" is *rachamim*, from the root *rechem* meaning "womb."

Is the dual nature of God hinted at in the Hebrew in the last line of Genesis 1:27, where the omission of the personal pronoun "He" suggests the reading "male and female created them"? The male and female aspects of God, God as *Elohim* and God as *Shechinah*, created the male and female forms of humankind. In the Hebrew we again have a plural subject, "male and female," and a singular verb, "created," echoing the plural form of God, *Elohim*, and the singular verbs "said" and "created" in these two verses.

God's creation of humankind in God's image is the fundamental fractal because each of us, born of dust, dying unto dust, bears the image of the Loving Mother-Father who creates us, the infinite, indefinable, beyond-all-words God, who is above all blessings and hymns and praises and consolations that are uttered in this world. But just as we need God, so does God need us. Only through humans could God learn how to balance justice and mercy, anger and love. Hence God's creation of humankind implies a reciprocity. God creates the human in God's image so that the human could create God in the human's image, two complementary and interdependent processes, each impossible without the other.

The first creation narrative, in which God is called *Elohim*, ends with God's resting on the seventh day. In the second creation narrative, God is called YHWH *Elohim*, often translated as the LORD God. This second narrative begins with God's creating the human anew from the dust of the earth, breathing into him the breath that in Genesis 1:2 was hovering over the waters. He "blew into his nostrils the breath of life, and the human became a living creature" (Gen. 2:7). No sooner is the human created than the duality principle, the defining principle of human existence, enters. Immediately we are told about the two trees in the Garden of Eden (Gen. 2:9) — the tree of life in the midst of the garden and the tree of knowledge of good and evil — and about the splitting of the river running out of Eden into four streams (Gen. 2:10–14).

Then God issued the fateful commandment to the man, not to the woman, who had not yet been created. "From the fruit of the garden you may surely eat. But from the tree of knowledge, good and evil, you shall not eat, for on the day you eat from it, you are doomed to die" (Gen. 2:16–17). Created from Adam's rib, the woman was then seduced by the serpent, or perhaps educated by it. She ate from the fruit and gave it to the man, who also ate. God confronted them, indicted them, punished them, and banished them from the garden. The banishment with which the dream narrative ends enunciates the fundamental duality of Jewish history: exile and redemption, a yin-yang of complementary and interdependent processes captured beautifully, as Benjamin Harshav points out, in the Hebrew wordplay, *golah* and *geulah*. Banishment from the garden is inseparable from the yearning to return.

This is the bare story, but the Garden of Eden narrative encompasses much more. Not only sin and sexual awakening, but also the birth of conceptual thinking and the development of self-consciousness through the acquisition of language. Also the resultant change in language from the sober, mathematical precision of science to the explosive, anxiety-ridden ambiguity of the emotions. The inevitable loss of innocence as humans mature. The suppression of the nurturing female by the aggressive male, first expressed in the birthing of the woman from the man in contradiction to the natural process of procreation (Gen. 2:21–22).

The insights given by the text into the nature of language are an aspect of its profundity. After creating the human, God spoke twice (Gen. 2:17–18), first to forbid the human from eating the fruit of the tree of knowledge of good and evil and then to announce God's intention "to make him a sustainer beside him." Adam became God's partner in creation. God did not name the creatures, but brought each one before Adam to see what he would call it, and that became the creature's name (Gen. 2:19). In this ceremony Adam the scientist articulated a mathematically precise mirror of reality that is devoid of shadow.

After Adam celebrated the birth of the woman in a two-line poem, chapter 3 and all the trouble begin. The serpent enters. During a meditation session that I led for graduate students in my department, one student related a story about a garter snake that had recently crossed her path at a bus stop. She bent down and talked to the snake, urging it to stay out of the way of an approaching bus. When she related this story to her grandfather, a traditional Southern Baptist, he replied that he would have acted differently. "That snake brought sin into the world, Paula. Read the Bible, chapter 3 of Genesis, verse 15. 'And I will put enmity between thee and the woman,' said God to the serpent. 'It shall bruise thy head, and thou shalt bruise his heel.' Paula, you should have stepped on it and crushed it before it bruises your head and worse."

I read the serpent differently, not as the bringer of sin into the world but as a wisdom-messenger of the messiness of life and the inherent ambiguity of language, which the serpent knows and must help Adam understand. In this regard he is a cousin of Satan, or the Prosecutor, in the Book of Job. In the first verse of that book, the main character is introduced as being *ish tam ve-yashar*, translated as "a man scrupulously moral" or more literally as "a man blameless and upright," the latter term reflecting the basic meaning of *yashar* as "straight." As we will explore in the next chapter, the role of the Prosecutor in the Book of Job is to teach Job to abandon the controlled, contrived artificiality of the *yashar* in order that he might embrace the curved, nonlinear, sinuous, and spontaneous explosiveness of life. In Adam's education in the garden, the roles of the serpent, of Eve, and, surprisingly, of God are similar. In order to become fully human, Adam must learn to speak the messy, imprecise language of the emotions.

A fascinating wordplay links the serpent and Eve, who are Adam's two best teachers. Called "the woman" through most of the Eden narrative, she is given her name Eve just before the expulsion. "And the human [Adam] called his woman's name Eve, for she was the mother of all that lives" (Gen. 3:20). This verse derives Eve's Hebrew name *Chavah* from a form of the Hebrew word *chai*, meaning "life." Robert Alter suggests another, intriguing possibility:

> It has been proposed that Eve's name conceals very different origins, for it sounds suspiciously like the Aramaic word for "serpent." . . . [M]ight there lurk behind the name a very different evaluation of the serpent as a creature associated with the origins of life?

As with Jacob, who is defined by duplicity and wordplay, a pun also introduces the serpent, about whom it is said that it was "most cunning of all the beasts of the field" (Gen. 3:1). The word translated as "cunning" is *arum*, the same term used to denote the nakedness of Adam and Eve in the preceding verse. "And the two of them were naked/*arumim*, the human and his woman, and they were not ashamed" (Gen. 2:25). Rashi picks up the sexual connotation, writing that the serpent "saw them unclothed, indulging in marital relations unashamedly, and he coveted her."

The text becomes opaque, a fractured, van Gogh nightmare-landscape where fruit is sex is concealment and self-consciousness is exile is redemption. The serpent addressed Eve, interpreting or twisting or manipulating God's words to the man commanding him not to eat from the tree of knowledge of good and evil. The serpent beguiled her to eat from the fruit of the tree. The woman ate, and she gave the fruit to her man, and he ate. Sexual awakening. Self-consciousness is born, as is the awareness of duality and separation. "And the eyes of the two were opened, and they knew they were naked, and they sewed fig leaves and made themselves loincloths" (Gen. 3:7).

Rashi makes the logical inference that the fruit they ate was a fig, confirming that there are no coincidences in the world of the spirit. Indeed, the Bodhi tree, the tree under which the Buddha meditated and attained enlightenment, was an Indian fig tree venerated as *ficus religiosa*. This cross-cultural connection invites us to view the drama in the garden through the lens of the Buddha's experience. Enlightenment is not possible in the pre-conceptual world preceding Eve's and Adam's eating the fig. They are us. Only after we learn concepts and then go beyond them, emptying ourselves of judgments, stories, analyses, and projections, will the fig and the tree on which it grows become the genesis of our own eventual enlightenment. After concepts have been transcended, our innate Buddha nature is given the space to bloom.

In the face of their sexual awakening, the birth of their self-consciousness, and their awareness of duality and separation, how did Adam and Eve respond? Not with jubilation, but as frightened human beings. They "hid from the LORD God in the midst of the trees of the garden" (Gen. 3:8). A potent moment in this drama now unfolds when God, the master of creation, innovates again, inventing a new, playful, almost flirtatious mode of discourse. "And the LORD God called to Adam and said to him, 'Where are you?' " (Gen. 3:9). Certainly God knew where Adam was. Perhaps God's open-ended question was meant to encourage Adam to reply in kind. My fascination with this potent moment of Adam's interaction with God was inspired by a 2004 lecture by Avivah Gottlieb Zornberg titled "Seduced into Eden: The Beginning of Desire." Several of the insights that I share in this discussion are due to her.

To God's question, "Where are you?", Adam answered, "I heard Your sound in the garden and I was afraid, for I was naked, and I hid" (Gen. 3:10). The response is momentous. Adam spoke about himself, the first act of self-reference by a human in the Hebrew Bible. Consciousness doubles back on itself to discover an independent ego-self. Self-consciousness creates the basic anxiety: I, the ego-laden subject, cut off from God, the source of all being. Agitated and fearful, Adam hid from himself and from God inside the fog of four I's. "I heard your sound in the garden and I was afraid, for I was naked, and I hid." This separation degenerates into the conflict and struggle expressed in God's punishment of Adam a few verses later (Gen. 3:17–19). "Cursed be the soil . . . with pangs shall you eat . . . [t]horn and thistle . . . sweat of your brow . . . for dust you are and to dust shall you return." The story ends as God drives Eve and Adam out of the garden, placing the flame of the whirling sword to guard the way to the tree of life (Gen. 3:24).

Adam's suffering when confronted by God in Genesis 3:9 reveals the existential truth, as Masao Abe explains in his book, *Zen and Western Thought*:

> Self-estrangement and anxiety are *not* something *accidental* to the ego-self, but are inherent to its structure.... To be human means to be an ego-self; to be an ego-self means to be cut off from both one's self and one's world; and to be cut off from one's self and one's world means to be in constant anxiety. This is the human predicament.

As we experience the drama of Eve and Adam in the garden, we confront the drama of our own suffering. Banished from Eden, separated by concepts from reality, from ourselves, and from the source of all being, we spend a lifetime trying to re-enter. How will we discover a new way of being unmediated by any conceptual lens?

The Buddha's answer is encapsulated in the Fourth Noble Truth, which is the way leading to the end of suffering. This way is the Noble Eightfold Path comprising right understanding, right intention, right speech, right action, right livelihood, right effort, right mindfulness, and right concentration. The last three qualities are cultivated by practicing meditation.

The Hebrew Bible also has an answer, not explicit like the Buddha's but encoded in the original Hebrew of Adam's response, the multidimensionality of which is completely obscured by translation. "I heard your sound in the garden and I was afraid, for I was naked, and I hid." This is only one of many interpretations of the original Hebrew, which explodes in the poetry of this verse.

The eleven words of the translation — "and I was afraid, for I was naked, and I hid" — are compressed in the original to a mere five: "*va-ira ki eyrom anochi va-eychave.*" The word *va-ira* corresponds to "and I was afraid," *ki* to "for," *eyrom* to "naked," *anochi* to I, and *va-eychave* to "and I hid." The second "was" is understood in the Hebrew original, which occasionally omits certain forms of the verb "to be." Hiding from himself and from God inside the fog of I's, Adam's pregnant phrase explodes into no less than twelve different readings, an emotional outburst signifying the depth of Adam's despair and the extent of Adam's confusion as his ego-self is born. It is no longer the articulation of sober, mathematical precision as when Adam named the animals. It is a creative, ambiguous, human outpouring that demands interpretation, as the rest of the Hebrew Bible does.

The twelve different readings arise because of the multiple meanings of the second, third, and fourth words in this verse. The word *ki*, translated here as "for," has numerous other meanings including "that." As we saw in verses 2:25 and 3:1, *eyrom*, like its variant *arum*, can be translated either as "naked" or as "cunning." Finally, as we saw in chapter 4 when we discussed Jacob's insight after his dream — "Indeed the Lord is in this place, and I did not know." (Gen. 28:16) — the fourth word, *anochi*, has three possible meanings: "I" or "ego" or "the Lord."

Corresponding to the two meanings of *ki*, the two meanings of *eyrom*, and the three meanings of *anochi*, the three-word phrase *ki eyrom anochi* in Genesis 3:10 has the sense of any of the following twelve readings. Each illuminates a different facet of Adam's state of mind at this breakthrough-moment of his life.

1) and I was afraid for I was naked, and I hid.
2) and I was afraid that I was naked, and I hid.
3) and I was afraid for my ego was naked, and I hid.
4) and I was afraid that my ego was naked, and I hid.
5) and I was afraid for God was naked, and I hid.
6) and I was afraid that God was naked, and I hid.
7) and I was afraid for I was cunning, and I hid.
8) and I was afraid that I was cunning, and I hid.
9) and I was afraid for my ego was cunning, and I hid.
10) and I was afraid that my ego was cunning, and I hid.
11) and I was afraid for God was cunning, and I hid.
12) and I was afraid that God was cunning, and I hid.

If we include the first and last Hebrew words — *va'ira*, translated as "I was afraid," and *va-eychave*, translated as "and I hid" — and the numerous other meanings of *ki*, then the possibilities mushroom further. In speaking these words, Adam is a linguistic innovator who introduces a specifically Biblical verb form, the *conversive vav*, that reverses past and future tenses. Specifically, the word *va-ira* consists of the verb *ira*, meaning "I will be afraid," preceded by *va*, which adds "and" and reverses the tense, yielding "and I was afraid"; similarly with *va-eychave*. However, since the Torah scroll has no vowels, we are also free to change the vowels in the first syllables of these words from *va* to *ve*, yielding "and I will be afraid" and "I will hide." As Avivah Gottlieb Zornberg pointed out in her 2004 lecture, the confusion of past and future expressed in Adam's words is a hallmark of human consciousness, which conceptualizes in a language that contaminates the past with the future and the future with the past.

The language of Adam's encounter with God in the garden and the themes involved in this encounter are echoed throughout the Hebrew Bible. This extraordinarily dense web of resonances has been amplified by more than 2000 years of exegesis. In a single chapter it is impossible to trace all the roots and repercussions, both linguistic and thematic, of this encounter and, in particular, of the exploding poetry of Genesis 3:10. We will finish by focusing on statement number 4 — "I was afraid that my ego was naked, and I hid" — an utterance having significant echoes in Buddhist thought.

According to Rabbi Hillel, the wisdom of the Hebrew Bible can be summarized in one teaching. Do not do unto others what you would not have them do unto you. The rest is commentary. According to the Buddha, his teachings can be summarized in one question. What is the cause of human suffering and how does one end it? Seeking an answer in the nature of the self, the Buddha taught that the self is a mental construct and that we suffer because we live under the illusion that the self is a fixed entity having an inner essence. As David Loy observes in *Lack and Transcendence: The Problem of Death and Life in Psychotherapy, Existentialism, and Buddhism*, this insight is related to the Freudian concept of repression:

> If our sense of self as something autonomous and self-grounded is a fiction, if the ego is in fact mentally constructed and socially internalized, then perhaps our primal repression is not sexual wishes (as Freud thought) nor fear of death (as many existential psychologists think) but the quite valid suspicion that *"I" am not real.*

When God confronted Adam in the garden, Adam replied, "I was afraid that my ego was naked, and I hid." Being exposed as naked before the truth can activate the process called in

Buddhism the Great Death, the process that brings one to the verge of solving the mystery of self. David Loy:

> Of course, if the sense-of-self is a construct — composed of automatized, mutually reinforcing ways of thinking, feeling and acting — it cannot really die, it can only evaporate in the sense that those cease to recur. Insofar as these constitute our basic psychological defenses against the world, however, this letting-go will not be easy. It means giving up my most cherished thoughts and feelings about myself (notice the reflexivity), *which are what I think I am*, to stand naked and exposed. Hence, Buddhism calls it the Great Death.

Another wordplay animates the Hebrew, giving yet another dimension to Adam's pregnant reply. We creatively transform the last word *va'eychave/*and I hid by changing several vowels, replacing the second letter *chet* by the letter *chaf*, which has the same sound, and replacing the silent last letter *aleph* by the silent letter *heh*. Then statement number 4 becomes "and I was afraid that my ego was naked, and I will extinguish [it] (*ve-achabeh*)" or "and I was afraid that my ego was naked, and I will be extinguished (*ve-echbeh*)." Perhaps Adam spoke, and God heard, one of these. By extinguishing my ego or by being extinguished, I die the Great Death of letting go of the illusion of the independent ego-self. These interpretations are energized by a potent word association that transcends language boundaries. The Buddhist term *nirvana*, the state of enlightenment free of all suffering, comes from a Sanskrit root meaning "to blow out" or "to extinguish."

Will Adam ever understand the implications of statement number 4? Will you? Will I? If so, then that statement is the grain of sand around which a pearl of wisdom can grow, leading him and you and me past the flame of the whirling sword back into the garden from which the ego-self banished itself. Then we will see, after a lifetime of struggle, that like the extinguished ego-self, you and I and the flame and the sword and the garden are mere concepts too. Our Buddha nature will unfold as the ultimate truth — that there is no ultimate truth — finally enlightens us.

6
Becoming Job: Going Beyond Words

> Were our mouth as full of song as the sea, and our tongue as full of joyous song as its multitude of waves, and our lips as full of praise as the breadth of the heavens, and our eyes as brilliant as the sun and the moon, and our hands as outspread as eagles of the sky and our feet as swift as hinds — we still could not thank You sufficiently, HASHEM our God and God of our forefathers, and to bless Your Name for even one of the thousand thousand, thousands of thousands and myriad myriads of favors that You performed for our ancestors and for us.
>
> "The Soul of Every Living Being,"
> *The Complete ArtScroll Siddur,* trans. Rabbi Nosson Scherman

DESPITE OUR STRIVING, or because of it, enlightenment eludes us. We are Eve and Adam at the end of chapter 3 of Genesis, banished from the Garden of Eden of our youth. Blind to our predicament, we wander fitfully, chasing shadows and mistaking them for wisdom. Our children fight. We are vulnerable and get sick. Surrounded by wonder, we grow old and suffer and die, the way back into our Garden of Eden blocked by our egos and our concepts.

Job could be our guide. Of all the books of the Hebrew Bible, his speaks the most eloquently about suffering, the search for justification, and spiritual growth. When pain afflicts us, we often act like Job, demanding explanations for our suffering and trying to rationalize it. But this doesn't bring peace. How can we find it? Will an inner voice of wisdom — our Buddha nature — reveal the truth, as did the voice of God that spoke to Job from the whirlwind? This voice will tell us that the way back into our Garden of Eden has always been just a breath away.

Of all the books of the Hebrew Bible, the Book of Job certainly speaks to me the most directly. From February 2000, when the headaches erupted, until the aftermath of my awakening in August 2003, I became Job. That my suffering followed the pattern of Job's I knew only too well. During the spring semester of 2000, while I trudged, helpless and vulnerable, from doctor to doctor begging for a cure, I was teaching a course at my university titled "Wrestling with the Book of Job: A Dialogue."

The Book of Job is one of the great outpourings of the human spirit. Written by an unknown, probably non-Jewish author in an unknown locale at an unknown period in history, the book reaches across the centuries to engage us in the paradoxes of suffering, evil, and the nature of God.

The story is famous. Job was "scrupulously moral, religious, one who avoided evil." The father of "seven sons and three daughters . . ., that man was one of the greatest people of the East."* The view shifts to the divine court, where God was challenged about Job's moral behavior by the Prosecutor, a translation of the Hebrew *hasatan*, often transliterated as "Satan." In response, God allowed the Prosecutor to destroy Job's flocks and kill his servants and his

---

* All translations from the Book of Job are taken from Edwin M. Good's *Turns of Tempest: A Reading of Job with a Translation*.

children. Yet Job refused to curse God. The Prosecutor challenged God again, and this time God allowed him to afflict Job's body with dreadful sores from the sole of his foot to the top of his head. Again, Job refused to curse God. But he cursed the day he was born; he demanded that God account to him for his sufferings; in his blindness to the truth, he casted God as his accuser, defender, and judge; he castigated God for being an immoral, nihilistic, voyeuristic thug; and he railed against his three friends, who came to torment Job with their simplistic moralizing.

When we suffer from physical or emotional pain, we often mimic Job by demanding to know. "What have I done to you, you watcher of men?" he shouts at God. "Why have you set me up as your target, so I've become a burden to myself?" (Job 7:20). With Job as our ventriloquist, we implore our family, friends, and doctors, "Why did this pain attack me? Why now? How long must I wait before I am healed?" "Don't condemn me," Job begs God. "Let me know of what you're accusing me" (Job 10:2). "Why me?" he screams. "Why me?" we echo. "I am neither tranquil nor quiet," Job complains, "and I have no rest; turmoil comes" (Job 3:26). "I am perfect — I don't know myself — I despise my life" (Job 9:21), he stammers.

Job's questions never received an answer. Our questions never receive an answer. They are the wrong questions. We don't even know the correct questions to ask. In perhaps the greatest poetry ever composed, God addressed Job from the whirlwind, describing the overwhelming splendor of nature that is infinitely beyond the capacity of the human mind to comprehend. Rejecting the simplistic, dualistic theology of Job's friends, God never addressed Job's demands for justice. "I transcend all concepts," God asserted. "They are the products of your impotent intellect. I incorporate both paradox and truth. Do not try to comprehend my ways." The book ends with God's restoring to Job double the possessions that he had before the catastrophe and bestowing upon Job and his wife seven new sons and three new daughters.

From the whirlwind God addressed Job with a poetry of blinding light and unfathomable depths that led to his enlightenment. On August 5, 2003, while I meditated in Barre, Massachusetts, a still, small voice whispered to me from the whirlwind of the suffering in which I had been lurching for more than three years. The voice whispered to me the truth about the pain.

What do we learn from the Book of Job? Certainly not that good people are rewarded and bad people are punished. Those views represent the conventional, concept-based moralizing of the friends, which God rebuffs. The spirituality of the book is much deeper and much more opaque. Among all the books of the Hebrew Bible, the Book of Job distinguishes itself by going beyond words and concepts, by insisting on the unfathomability of pain and adversity and on the cognitive and moral abyss between humans and God. According to the Job-poet, pain and adversity cannot be figured out and rationalized, the tragedies of life and the infinite wonders of nature cannot be captured by a coherent narrative. One can either reject the mystery or open up to it with a reverent silence and a sense of wonder. Concerning the meaning of the Book of Job, Edwin M. Good writes the following at the end of his 400-page commentary, the fruit of a career devoted to this text: ". . . I come to the end of my reading of Job with the conviction that the book remains open and multiple, its 'meaning' indeterminate and undecidable. . . ."

The indeterminacy of the Book of Job works not only on the level of the text but also on the level of individual words. An illuminating example occurs in the following five verses, which appear in the first two chapters (my italics):

> Perhaps my children have *blessed* Elohim *sinfully* in their hearts. (Job 1:5)
> [Y]ou . . . *blessed* anything his hands do. . . . (Job 1:10)
> If he doesn't *curse* you to your face — (Job 1:11)
> Yahweh's name be *blest*. (Job 1:21)
> *Curse* Elohim and die! (Job 2:10)

I was certainly surprised to learn that each of the italicized phrases and words — blessed sinfully, blessed, curse, blest, curse — are translations of Hebrew words having the identical root *b-r-ch*, traditionally translated as "bless." Although blessing and cursing are central to the text, motivating much of the book's dialogue, in most cases it is not clear which of the two senses of these apparently opposite concepts are intended. Edwin M. Good extrapolates from this indeterminacy to a way of approaching the entire book:

> [My goal is] to help readers liberate their imaginations, wherever the word appears, to focus on its depth, not on its shallowness, on its multiplicity, not its illusory simplicity. The very centrality of *brk* [sic] prevents smug certainty that we know the meaning of this story.

The multiplicity of meanings of this single root suggests that bless/curse, and by extension all dualistic thinking, do not represent opposites but point to something much more profound. They are dynamic word-clusters involving complementary and interdependent processes, much like Indra's Net in Buddhist thought. In the same way that we read the Book of Job, focusing on its depth and the multiplicity of its meanings, so may we live our lives, particularly when, like Job, pain and suffering afflict us.

Although the ultimate meaning of the Book of Job is opaque, the text hints why Job was singled out for punishment. The first verse tells us that Job was scrupulously moral and religious, a man of perfect integrity, blameless and upright. But he was religious to a fault, fearing the penalties of sin, anticipating sin even before it happened:

> . . . Job would sanctify them [his children], getting up early in the morning and offering sacrifices for each one. For Job said, "Perhaps my children have blessed Elohim sinfully in their hearts." (Job 1:5)

A small-minded piety seems to motivate Job, who is caught in the prison of dualistic thinking: blessing versus curse, morality versus sin, reward versus punishment. Job will suffer because he will bang his head against the walls of this conceptual prison until he is bruised and bloody. Only after God's speech from the whirlwind opened his eyes to see that the prison of dualistic thinking is an illusion could Job liberate himself.

It could be only Job's unstable and petty religiosity that brought him to the attention of God, who in turn brought him to the attention of the Prosecutor, tempting the Prosecutor to test Job's piety:

> "Have you given thought to my servant Job? There's no one like him on the earth, a scrupulously moral man, religious, one who avoids evil." (Job 1:8)

Interestingly, the word translated here as "servant" could also be translated as "slave." The Prosecutor took notice of God's servant/slave Job, and then Job's ordeal began.

Another irony links my life with Job. Not only was I teaching a course on the Book of Job during the springtime of my headaches, but also, about a month after the headaches had erupted, I gave a talk on Job that was outwardly humorous, inwardly right on the mark concerning Job's shortcomings — and my own.

The occasion of the talk was the annual Latke Versus Hamantash Debate, sponsored by Hillel House at the University of Massachusetts Amherst. The purpose of the debate is to argue the merits of two traditional foods for the Jewish holidays: the latke, a pancake made out of grated potatoes and eaten during Chanukah, versus the hamantash, a triangular cake filled with prunes and eaten during Purim. In the great debate of March 2000 I took the side of the latke and created the latke code. Simultaneously tongue-in-cheek and insightful, the code reveals spiritual truths about Job and through Job, about myself.

Consider the different recipes. *The Great Hadassah WIZO Cookbook* tells us that to make hamantashen, one cuts the dough into rounds and squares, pinches the rounds into triangles, and folds the squares over the triangle. Notice the degree of human control: cut, pinch, fold. On the shaping of the hamantashen we impose an overarching human will. Cut. Pinch. Fold. The recipe for latkes is much simpler. One merely drops the potatoes and onions, eggs and seasoning and matzo meal into the hot pan and lets the laws of nature and of God determine the shape.

The difference is clear. The hamantash represents the artificial, the controlled, the non-spontaneous. The latke represents what is authentic, impetuous, and spontaneous, submitting itself to the profound shaping-laws of nature and of God rather than to the artificial shaping by mere human hands. As such, it is a culinary vessel containing the Buddha's wisdom about life.

As explained on the website of Dictionary.com Unabridged, etymology also reveals the superiority of the latke, linguistically mirroring the peregrinations of the Jewish people. *Latke* is a Yiddish word derived from the Ukrainian *oladka* after wandering diminutively through Old Russian as *olad'ya*, where it arrived after crossing northeast from the Greek *eladia*, plural of *eladion*, meaning "little oily thing." We trace *eladion* back to a diminutive of *elaion*, meaning "olive oil," ultimately to *elaiā*, meaning "olive," the most noble nectar of the Mediterranean terrain.

With its roots sunk deep in Jewish mythology — "And the dove came back to him at eventide and look, a plucked olive leaf was in its bill, and Noah knew that the waters had abated from the earth." (Gen. 8:11) — the olive became the symbol of Athena, who planted the first olive tree on Greek soil. Appropriately, the god in charge of the care of olive trees is Hermes, whose representative in the Hebrew Bible is Jacob. The fruit of the olive tree nourishes the body, gives light, and heals wounds and all manner of human woes. Its branches crown heroes' heads and, when the end comes, accompanies the souls of the dead across the River Acheron to Hades on Charon's doleful boat. In order to immortalize the link between the latke and the noble olive, the sun under which the olive tree thrives has the shape of the latke, the Greek gods' bequest to the Jewish people.

By contrast, the hamantash is etymologically flat. *Hamantash* is a Yiddish word meaning "Haman's pocket," which presumably refers to the shape of the cake. Haman was the Persian minister whose thwarted plot to murder the Jews of Shushan is recorded in the Book of Esther and is celebrated at Purim.

The Hebrew language also confirms the ascendancy of the latke over its rigidly triangular, prune-filled rival. As we have seen, the word is the beloved great-granddaughter of the Greek word for olive, which in Hebrew is *zayit*, which rhymes with *bayit*, which means house, which evokes the warm ambience in which latkes are savored. By contrast, the Hebrew phrase for hamantashen is *ozney Haman*, meaning "Haman's ears." Who would want to eat those? Spiritually, etymologically, as well as culinarily, the hamantash is an indigestible dead end.

One never sees a straight line in nature. Transferring this observation from the natural world to the culinary world, one never sees hamantashen in nature, only latkes, in the shape of the moon and the sun, for example. This has everything to do with the Book of Job, for if we decode the beginning of the book using the latke code, we discover that Job's favorite food was the hamantash, for which he had a mad obsession. And this obsession led to his downfall.

The Book of Job opens with this: "Once there was a man in the country of Uz named Job, a man *tam ve-yashar* / scrupulously moral, religious, one who avoided evil." I will pass over the influence of Job's Uz upon Dorothy-of-Kansas's Oz. Rather, I focus on the Hebrew phrase *tam ve-yashar*. Translated here as "scrupulously moral," this phrase can be rendered more literally as "blameless and upright." In the words of the Chinese fortune cookie that Job serendipitously received, "you have a reputation for being honest and straightforward." The word *tam*, meaning "innocent" or "blameless" or even "simple," has another connotation in Book of Job, echoing the Hebrew word and the Yiddish word for "taste." Since the next Hebrew word *yashar* means literally "straight," the latke code interprets *tam ve-yashar* as "a taste for the straight," which can only mean that

Job loved the straight, humanly controlled, artificial shape of the hamantash.

This is borne out by the first illustration of William Blake for the Book of Job, which depicts Job and his family sitting in rigidly vertical positions.* The latke-shapes of the sun and the pale moon on the horizon and of the musical instruments on the tree above Job's head symbolize enlightenment. But Job does not notice them. He stares mechanically straight ahead as his hand grasps the edges of a book of law, which he seems about to pinch and fold into the triangular shape of his favorite, *tam ve-yashar* food.

Further evidence that the hamantash leads to Job's downfall comes in the first speech of the Prosecutor to God. "Is Job religious for nothing? Haven't you yourself hedged around him and his family and all he has, blessed anything his hands do. . .?" (Job 1:9–10). The key words here are "hedged" and "hands," both of which start with the letter H, the first letter of Job's favorite food. The meaning is clear. God has hedged Job in with a human-hand-shaped hamantash.

Inadvertently, Job picks up the cue in his first long speech when he talks of God hedging around him, using images that connote blockage and restriction: darkness, thick gloom, blackness, belly, womb, prison, burial mound, grave (Job 3:5–23). Job is not facing the truth. He is being hedged around not by God but by the hamantash of his own constricted ego, which actualizes its worst fears. "For I was terrified of something, and it arrived, what I fear comes to me" (Job 3:25).

---

* William Blake's illustrations for the Book of Job can be viewed at *http://www.bc.edu/bc_org/avp/cas/ashp/blake_job_text.html*.

The latke code also reveals a deep correspondence between the Book of Job and Franz Kafka's novel, *The Trial*. This correspondence builds on the observation of Gershom Scholem, the great scholar of Jewish mysticism whom Kafka deeply influenced. In his essay on Kafka, Robert Alter points out that not only do the plots of both books center on what Scholem calls a "secret trial," but also for Scholem "Kafka's novel is a profound and authentic new expression, perhaps the first in two and a half millennia, of the radical theology of Job."

The latke code reveals the secret meaning of Kakfa's sketch in the first chapter of an edition of his novel that I have. As the chapter opens, Job's modern counterpart, Josef K., learns that he is being arrested for a crime that is never revealed (notice the "JO" sound linking Job and Josef). Kafka's sketch shows Josef K. being hedged in by a triangular lattice having the shape of a hamantash, allowing us to deduce Josef K.'s crime. Like his Biblical precursor, he prefers the hamantash's rigidly straight philosophy over the latke's going-with-the-flow spontaneity. Job eventually sees the truth. Tragically, Josef K. does not. He dies by the straight edge of a knife thrust deep into his *tam ve-yashar* heart and turned there twice.

Now a fundamental question arises. Where does the latke make its first appearance in the Book of Job? Because the latke represents what is natural and spontaneous, you will not be surprised that the latke is the symbol of the Prosecutor, whose challenges to God lead to Job's suffering and ultimately Job's enlightenment. As we learn from Blake, everything in Job's world is straight and hamantash-like while everything in the spiritual realm floating over Job's head is curved and latke-like, foremost the Prosecutor, who stretches undulatingly and sinuously between the two domains. Blake depicts the same latke-motif in another illustration showing the Prosecutor going forth from the presence of the Lord to "strike Job with dreadful sores from the sole of his foot to the top of his head" (Job 1:7).

The latke code reveals the secret. The Prosecutor's goal was to teach Job not to be straight and not to be *yashar*, not to approach the world using the rigid philosophy of the hamantash based on willfulness and control. The Prosecutor's goal was to teach Job to circumvent, to go around, to go with the flow of the latke as he learned to act spontaneously. An advantage of living in the modern era is that we can read the spiritual truth — although most of us are blind to its message — in *The Great Hadassah WIZO Cookbook*, which instructs us not to shape the latke at all, but merely to drop the divine delectation of potatoes and onions, eggs and seasoning and matzo meal into the hot pan and let the laws of nature and of God determine the shape. Job did not have such a book. He had to learn the hard way.

In chapter 38, God answered Job from the whirlwind. Of all places from which to answer Job, the whirlwind is the least straight, the least *yashar*, the least hamantash-like. As illustrated by Blake, in a whirlwind there are only curves and loops, crescents and curls; all is complexly and interlockingly and fractally interwoven. A whirlwind is the most latke-like locus in God's creation. Here God revealed to Job the secret of life. In the words of Robert Alter, it is "a vision of outrageous and unwarranted human suffering, . . . of an unfathomable and cruelly beautiful nature that denies all the comforts of anthropocentrism," of the human-centered hamantash-philosophy of Job and his friends.

As God is about to answer Job from the whirlwind, Job's hands are in an attitude of supplication. "Please forgive me for trying to shape life like a hamantash. Teach me to go with the flow of life like a latke." And this is what God's poetry spoken from the whirlwind does. Finally, Job understood, and he answered God thus (Job 42:3, 5–6):

> "Therefore I told, and didn't understand,
> wonders beyond me, and I didn't know.
> ....
> With ears' hearing I hear you,
> and now my eye sees you.
> Therefore I despise and repent
> of dust and ashes."

To "repent of dust and ashes" is to reject the conventional understanding of society, which tries to explain the world in terms of concepts such as guilt and innocence. This is Job's enlightenment: to realize, as Edwin M. Good observes, that "the issue of repentance and the admission of sin . . . is the wrong issue. That structure of guilt and innocence was the focus of the friends' arguments. But the world spins on its own kind of order, of which Job had very little sense." To "repent of dust and ashes" is thus to go beyond words and concepts. It is to give up knowing. It is to embrace life as an open-ended, unfathomable mystery — as symbolized by the latke — without reducing it to the constricted confines of human logic — as symbolized by the hamantash.

Blake ends his illustrations of the Book of Job by showing Job and his family playing the musical instruments that in the first illustration had been hanging on the tree right above Job's head. In a paraphrase of Moses (Deut. 30:12–14), insight is not in the heavens and is not beyond the sea, but is very close to Job, just an arm's length away. Having attained enlightenment after he heard God speak from the whirlwind,

Job celebrated the latke-shapes of the instruments and of the sun and the moon on the horizon. Finally, the illusions of his old hamantash-way of living dissolved.

As the latke code reveals, the Book of Job is a record of Job's spiritual, culinary, and geometric transformations. He learned to abandon the straight, controlled lines of the hamantash in favor of the spontaneous curves of the latke. However, something has been lost between Job's time and ours. Although Job learned the multiple lessons of the latke, we have forgotten it. In our egocentric, technological civilization, the hamantash has again taken the ascendancy. We still live by its rigid, geometric laws, thinking that we can control the flow of life when in fact we are swimming in its infinite stream. Throw away your hamantashen, everyone. Learn the law of the latke. Life is curved, not straight. Don't try to cut and shape and pinch your life. Do as *The Great Hadassah WIZO Cookbook* says. Merely drop the divine delectation of potatoes and onions, eggs and seasoning and matzo meal into the hot pan and let the laws of nature and of God determine the shape.

This is what I talked about on that afternoon in March 2000. But the person to whom it should have spoken most deeply — me — was not ready for its message. Like Job, I was living by the rigid, geometric laws of the hamantash, deluded that I could control the flow of life when in fact I was swimming in its infinite stream. Life is curved, not straight, I said about Job, but it was all in the head, not in the heart. That day, I charted the course of my own healing, but it would take years before I could decode my own code.

7
What Pain Can Teach Us

> [W]e should begin practicing the teaching of the Buddha now because life is short and its end is unpredictable. The Buddha set forth three more reasons why we should act now:
> Rare is birth as a human being.
> Scarce is the probability of hearing the Dharma.
> Serious is the delusion of our mind.
> — Buddhas.net <*http://www.buddhas.net/when.html*>

HEADACHE PAIN HAS BEEN my best teacher. Physical or emotional pain can also become your best teacher, becoming a path to verifying the truth of Buddhist teachings. In order to inspire you to reexamine your experiences with suffering and pain, in this chapter I weave together personal narratives, experiences while meditating, medical reports, and insights into the suffering I had brought upon myself by trying to push the pain away. This suffering was healed when after years of anger and cursing, I finally faced the pain and accepted it without judgment and without commentary.

If you have suffered from illness or pain, then perhaps my experiences will resonate with you. Such suffering is but one path into the garden of Buddhist wisdom. It is an aspect of the suffering that the Buddha saw as symptomatic of the human condition. He taught that if one tries to understand the world in a conventional way, then suffering is inevitable. Joseph Goldstein explains the source of this suffering in his Dharma talk on the life of the Buddha:

> Conventional understanding of the world can be expressed in two words. And these are the words "to have." We have possessions. We have relationships. We have professions. We have a mind. We have a body. Our world is constructed within this framework of having. . . . But there's a problem in this. And the problem inherent in this worldview of having is that because of the great truth of impermanence and change, there is nothing that we have that we won't lose. . . . This truth of change is happening on every level that we look. Whatever we have eventually will be lost. So always in the world of having there is always an underlying, and sometimes very subtle, sense of unease or uncertainty or insecurity or incompleteness.

The Buddha used the term *dukkha* to refer to suffering from illness and pain as well as to this "sense of unease or uncertainty or insecurity or incompleteness." In this more generalized sense, *dukkha* arises because nothing lasts and everything changes, not only material possessions but also bodies, mental states, relationships, experiences, entire civilizations and cultures. Refusing to accept this universal truth of impermanence and change, we grasp at the impermanent, hoping that it will stay fixed, and when it inevitably does not, we suffer.

As the headaches have taught me to do, open yourself up to the *dukkha* in your life with mindful silence and perfect trust in the wisdom of your body, of the universe, of the present moment. That wisdom will reveal itself to you when it is ready.

Two levels of my basic insight

Level 1. My pain has led me to see that the truth is in my pain.

Level 2. My pain has led me to see that the pain does not exist. It is a conceptual abstraction. There is no pain, only energy flow and energy blockage.

Medication and meditation. Meditation is not a substitute for medical treatment and medication. However, in my experience medication and meditation were two divergent paths.

My experience with medication: alleviation of symptoms through chemicals; quick relief; harmful side effects; changed personality; dependence upon chemicals and upon doctors; no wisdom.

My experience with meditation: alleviation of symptoms through insight; an all-encompassing, artful approach to my entire life; end of suffering; healing myself; wisdom.

Medication erected an impregnable wall around my pain that wisdom could not enter. Meditation was more than a door that let the wisdom in. It showed me that the wall was a conceptual illusion.

A day with my teacher. After a stress-free and pain-free day, I wake up from a deep sleep at 2:13 AM with a pain in my nose.

Pain is a concept. There is no pain, only the sensation of tightness pinching the bridge of my nose as I finally fall asleep again. When I wake up in the morning, the tightness has almost vanished. I meditate, first analyzing the tightness and causing it to congeal into a solid mass. Then I just observe. The mass melts and flows into my forehead and back into the middle of the nose. No suffering, only noting the sensation, both while meditating and while working. In the mid-afternoon I take a short rest. Again the tightness flows as soon as I shut my eyes. After five minutes I get up refreshed, the tightness still there, ebbing and flowing, moving and churning. No problem. No suffering. Thus a day in March 2005.

In December 2000 the experience was different. Here is a passage from chapter 2 of this book describing my suffering:

> I find a comfortable chair and shut my eyes and follow my breath, noting that the pain isn't bad today, just a wave of sensation rolling between my eyes. Breath in. Breath out. Breath in, getting caught in the wave, which becomes angry and surges down the damaged nerve into my nasal passage — I can't stop it although I know what is about to happen — and transmogrifies there into the sharp, pinching clamped-plier-throbbing-pressure of nose pain that is so sharp that following my breath mindfully becomes as impossible as excising my nose from my face, which I'd really like to do because it hurts so fucking bad.

What changed between December 2000 and March 2005? The perception of pain was still there, but the suffering was gone. No story, no drama, no expectations. The pain comes, the pain goes, "illusory appearances," in the words of Lama Tashi Namgyal, "lacking any substantial reality":

> From the standpoint of ultimate truth, all phenomena, including all the phenomena that we misapprehend as physical matter, are empty of any inherent existence. Though they appear to be very solid and real to us, they are in truth mere illusory appearances lacking any substantial reality, like a light show in space, like the aurora borealis, a rainbow, an echo, a flash of lightning, a mirage, a magical display, a dream, an hallucination, like the images in movies and on television, or like the reflection of the moon in water.

The pain has enabled me to glimpse the nature of reality. Blessed be the pain.

When the pinching nose-pain decides to spend the day with me, I observe that the pressure on my nose equals the pressure of gravity on my butt when I'm sitting or the pressure of gravity on my feet when I'm walking. When the pinching pain spends the day with me, I imagine that I'm sitting on my nose or walking on my nose.

Analyzing the pain. Until the truth revealed itself at the meditation retreat in August 2003, the pinching nose-pain just described in the passage from December 2000 drove me crazy. Tormented by it whenever it appeared, for two years I tried to correlate the pain with the stress level of the previous day. Here are typical entries in my pain-diary:

March 17, 2002. Quiet day yesterday. Woke up 4 am clear-headed. Then had a dream I couldn't remember. Woke up again with nose pain. Lasted all day except for about an hour after lunch.

March 21, 2002. Worked all day and into the evening on the math paper. Why am I having so much trouble writing it? I couldn't fall asleep. Took sleeping pill at midnight, woke up 1:30 AM with nose pain. Lasted all day.

March 23, 2002. Again very relaxed yesterday except when Alison said something about my novel that almost got to me, but didn't. Woke up 1 AM with the nose pain, fell asleep but slept poorly. The pain lasted all day, throbbing.

March 27, 2002. Had a nice day working at home yesterday and a super dinner that Alison made. Pain at 2 AM. Sleeping pill. Up at 7 AM miraculously pain-free. The guys came to refinish the floors and stressed me out. The pinching nose-pain erupted. Nap at noon. Pain disappeared. Stressful email from my department head — "Richard, we need you to serve on the Personnel Committee next year." — and the pain returned.

I could never figure it out. The pinching nose-pain visited me with the same frequency and the same intensity both after relaxing days and after stressful days. After the 2003 meditation retreat, I stopped keeping a pain-dairy. It was time to give up knowing.

Theorems in the calculus of pain. During the first year of the headaches, early in my experience with the pinching nose-pain, I formulated the following three theorems:

> Theorem 1. If the pain is in my nose in the morning, then it will stay all day.
>
> Theorem 2. The pain always vanishes after a night's sleep.
>
> Theorem 3. Although meditating in the morning sometimes causes the pain to appear, this never happens in the afternoon or evening.

All three theorems have proved to be false.

Blaming myself and others for the headaches. Am I to blame for the headaches? Is anyone? My inability to figure out what causes the nose pain to appear on any given day is a pale planet orbiting the sun of a more dazzling unknowability. What complex chain of conditions caused the headaches to begin in February 2000? Melissa's wedding; disagreeing with my wife about the wedding; the plethora of perceived rejections: 1997 math book, National Science Foundation grant, prestigious university fellowship, my children growing up, my father; a genetic predisposition to headaches; my life experiences and those of my parents and my parents' parents and my parents' parents' parents, all the way back to Eve and Adam; the life experiences of every being in the universe, an intricately interwoven web of interrelations in which my headaches are just one of infinitely many threads? Are my headaches rooted in Eve's and Adam's trauma of being evicted from the garden and then learning that their elder son killed their younger son?

Am I to blame for the headaches? Is anyone? What causes the nose pain to appear? What caused the headaches to begin? Though grammatically correct, these strings of words shed their meaning, like a serpent its skin, when examined under the blinding light of the Great Unknowable.

Blame and causality: concepts that constrict consciousness. Lovingkindness and forgiveness open it up.

Suffering from the books I have written. On May 25, 2007, while our daughter Melissa and her husband were away on vacation, Alison and I stayed in their New York City apartment to celebrate my sixtieth birthday. But the celebration was marred by a loud, beeping noise that kept us up all night. It wasn't the smoke detector, and it wasn't the carbon monoxide detector, and by the time I had excluded these two possibilities, it was too late to call Melissa to ask her. In the morning we did. "Oh, it was my beeper," she answered. "Why didn't you shut it off?"

I couldn't control the beeper, and despite my best attempts I can't control life. In April 2003, a literary agent sent me an email after reading an essay of mine on my personal web page. "I've started a literary agency," she wrote, "in part hoping to help brilliant and literate scholars develop highly marketable properties." Her email was the seed from which the present book grew, a book nurtured and pruned and nourished by the agent's loving care. The tenth draft was completed in the spring of 2007, ready for submission to publishers. On May 22, 2007, three days before the beeper experience in Melissa's apartment, the literary agent informed me that for personal reasons she was closing her agency and could no longer represent the book. "Why are you abandoning me now?" I thought. "We are almost in the promised land."

The books I have written, of which the present book is the fourth, have caused me to suffer, each in its own way.

In 1985 I published my first math book. It caused me great suffering because I obsessed about errors that might have demolished its conceptual structure like a house of cards. But being a math book, it could not heal the suffering that it had caused.

So I wrote a novel, in which the suffering caused by the math book was a major theme. But I couldn't publish the novel, which caused me great suffering because publication had become my only goal. Although it was a novel and not a math book, the novel did not heal the suffering that it had caused.

In 1997 I published a second math book with Paul Dupuis. I loved working with him. But the book did not bring us recognition, which again caused me great suffering. And again this math book could not heal the suffering that it had caused.

So I got headaches and wrote this book, in which the suffering caused by the two math books and by the novel, compounded by the suffering caused by the headaches, are a major theme. When in May 2007 the literary agent told me that she could no longer represent this book, I suffered. When I spent the next two years seeking a publisher, I suffered. But this book turned out to be different from the first three. Through the process of writing it, the headaches have become my best teacher, instructing me how to use meditation and Buddhist teachings to deal with suffering. Finally, I had written a book that healed the suffering that it had caused.

What happened with the beeper in Melissa's apartment, with the literary agent, and with my four books reflects the present book's deep message: life is the play of impersonal forces that one can observe without getting sucked in.

Meditation is a door into pain. After the August 2003 retreat at the Insight Meditation Society, I didn't return for another three years. Did I need three years to assimilate the insights? Was I afraid? In August 2006 I was back for more wisdom, staying in a room that I had handpicked three years earlier. It seemed to be as close to perfection as possible: off the corridor, carpeted, pleasantly asymmetric, far away from the bathroom, a view of the woods. What I had not anticipated was that, despite our immersion in meditation, one or more of the nearby occupants would have door-slamming fetishes that, like Dracula, came out only when the sun was down, the closer to midnight the better. I limped through every night of the retreat with fractured sleep, but rather than complain, I tried to make this experience part of the practice.

Such equanimity was particularly hard on the next-to-last night when I went to bed at 9:40, was awakened by a slamming door around 10:30, fell asleep, was startled into wakefulness by another slamming door and by noise that continued past midnight, fell asleep, up at 4:30 with tightness and pinching pressure at the top of the nose. Full-fledged nose-pain greeted the rising sun. What to do? Anger would only make it worse, but there was no anger. The door slammers had no intention to harm me. I said to myself, "Welcome, pain. Thank you for giving me the opportunity to put into practice what I've learned on this retreat." As I write this, my openness surprises me.

At the 8:15 AM sitting we were urged again to let go of thoughts. The teacher, Anna Douglas, cited a recent study at Stanford University which revealed that the average person has some 63,000 thoughts a day and that of these, ninety-four percent are repetitive. "Nothing is worth thinking about," she said. "Pay attention not to the content of thoughts, but to the process of thinking. How it feels, and how effortlessly the mind knows. How sounds just appear, with no effort on our part. How the breath breathes itself, with no effort on our part. How bodily sensations arise, with no effort on our part. They are all on the same level."

I listen to her words and pay attention. The sky is blue, the clouds big, the world green, a breeze. Just thoughts. I come in contact with the sensation in my nose. A solid block of pain. I enter it, and the pain dissolves into a two-beat pulsing, which I enter, and it decomposes into a multi-beat fluttering, each with a different texture. And when I enter that, it deconstructs into a dance of microscopic, shimmering palpitations, a mirage, a jewel in the sun, a pond caressed by a breeze. Thoughts. I'm thinking. There's no pain, no I, no blame, no regret, no doors, only the shimmering, unfolding fractal of energy, each layer more intricate and microscopic than the one before, an inverted Jacob's ladder with its head approaching the earth, garden, trees, grass, branches, twigs, ants wearing twinkling anklets playing an infinitesimal music softer than a flower opening.

Astonished, I opened my eyes. Never before had I sensed such depth and texture in the nose pain, each layer revealing yet a deeper level of ever finer micro-processes, occurring and changing moment to moment, evanescent, fluttering, a spiderweb of fluctuating feeling. This, I realized, is what the practice is about. To sense reality as it is. There is no pain. That's just a label. There is no solid block of sensation. That illusion vanishes only when we are able to sense the gaps within the sensation. On the level of moment-to-moment awareness, it's all energy dancing in my face. It jumps, flickers, effervesces, stiffens, relaxes, twists, flares up, extinguishes itself, and returns, forever transforming.

During a walk in the woods on the day after I returned home, I saw the same dance of energy as the leaves fluttered in the breeze. The energy of my face. The energy of the universe, which Mu Soeng Sonim describes in his book, *Heart Sutra: Ancient Buddhist Wisdom in the Light of Quantum Reality*:

> Energy, whether of wave or particle, is associated with activity, with dynamic change. Thus the core of the universe — whether we see it as the heart of the atom or our own consciousness — is not static but in a state of constant and dynamic change. This energy — now wave, now particle — infuses each and every form at the cellular level. No form exists without being infused by this universal energy; form and energy interpenetrate each other endlessly in an ever-changing dance of the molecules, creating our universe.

Medical hell. The headaches erupted in February 2000. Panicked by the severity of the pain, its appearance from out of nowhere, the absence of a definitive diagnosis, and my inability to get to the bottom of it, I took action: an MRI of the brain and consultations with a number of doctors. In so doing, I created my own hell, panic compounded by uncertainty compounded by the feeling, which I got from every doctor but one, that I was a machine, not a human being.

The only exception was Dr. Nagagopal Venna, a neurologist at the Massachusetts General Hospital whose kindness and support contributed to my healing.

Here are paraphrased excerpts from six medical reports from the first half-year of the headaches together with excerpts from Dr. Venna's first report in July 2000 and his second report in February 2003. The diagnoses I received were as follows: facial dysesthesiae diathesis, mild sinus disease, low-grade migraine-type constitutional dysregulation, cluster headaches, stress-related tension headaches, vidian neuralgia, atypical form of migraine, atypical facial pain with neuralgic features, a variation of trigeminal neuralgia. No wonder I was confused.

Neurologist's report in March 2000. The neurologist found the neurological examination to be within normal limits. It did not indicate any pyramidal tract dysfunction, myelopathy, radiculopathy, or neuropathy. The main differential diagnosis of my headache or facial dysesthesiae diathesis is mild sinus disease versus tension. My sensitivity to lights and perfume suggests a low-grade, migraine-type constitutional dysregulation.

MRI of the brain in March 2000. The report states that images of the brain were obtained using previously mentioned pulse sequences. There is no enlargement of the ventricular system, and no areas of abnormal, increased or decreased signal are seen in the cerebral or cerebellar hemispheres. The MRI does not reveal any findings characteristic of hemorrhage or infarction, and no mass effect is visualized. The MRI does reveal a small, 7 mm rounded shadow in the anterior right maxillary antrum that could reflect a small area of inflammatory disease in the right maxillary sinus. Correlation with clinical findings in this area is recommended.

Primary care physician's report in April 2000. The doctor stated that I was seen for follow-up and review of my complex problem of highly atypical headaches manifesting as nose pain. He also mentioned that the MRI shows some questionable sinus disease and that I have been completing a course of Doxycycline, the effectiveness of which has been unclear. The doctor reported that my headaches continue and that I feel that anxiety about my daughter's upcoming wedding is a contributing factor.

Otolaryngologist's report in June 2000. The doctor reported that he is unsure why I am having my symptoms. Although my headaches seem directly related to stress, the symptoms seem to fit a pattern that would be similar to cluster headaches.

The otolaryngologist recommended that I take the medication Klonapin, which would have strong side effects.

Another neurologist's report in June 2000. This neurologist wrote that my problem is difficult. If it is not referred from local pathology, then nasal pain might suggest a diagnosis of vidian neuralgia, which could be referred from neck spasm. He went on to say that I am stubborn that it throbs, which suggests that this may be some atypical form of migraine or so-called lower half headache.

I decoded his saying I was "stubborn" to mean that my symptoms could not be pigeonholed in the neurologist's orderly conceptual universe.

Dr. B.'s report in June 2000. Dr. B. reported that I am experiencing atypical facial pain with neuralgic features. He increased Tegretol to Tegretol-XR 200 mg b.i.d. and advised that a week after I taper off Amitriptyline, I should begin to taper Clonazepam by 0.25 mg every third day and stop it also. Dr. B. asked me to keep pain diaries and to return to see him for another evaluation in one month.

Because the decreased medication was accompanied by greatly increased discomfort, Dr. B. soon loaded me with drugs, including Nortriptyline and others. My appointment with him on September 1, 2000 was unique among all my interactions with doctors for its complete breakdown in communication, and I stopped seeing him. He took his revenge by writing a sarcastic letter to my primary care physician, a letter predated June 29, 2000 and filled with inaccuracies, innuendoes, and amateur psychologizing that I allowed to make the headaches worse. Although I wanted to respond with my own angry letter, Melissa advised me not to. "Let it go, Dad," she said, sage counsel from a wise woman. Letting go became one of the central themes of my eventual healing.

Dr. Nagagopal Venna's first report in July 2000. In this report Dr. Venna wrote the following. "His wife . . . does say that while he was on these medications she has noticed a definite change in his mood and behavior, although the patient states that he does not feel depressed, sad, or hopeless. He does say that he tends to cry more easily than before. The wife has noticed that he has become quieter in his behavior, and the wife says that there is certainly a clear change in his normally vivacious behavior. . . . The constellation of symptoms do suggest a neuralgia in the distribution of some branches of the trigeminal nerve and has some features of sphenopalatine neuralgia. . . . I would consider this as a variation of a trigeminal neuralgia. . . . My expectation is that it will gradually get better over the next few months spontaneously."

In the winter of 2003 I started to meditate daily. Here is Dr. Venna's second report, in which he encouraged me to rely more on relaxation and meditation to control the pain rather than on drugs. Within a few months, I would reduce my drug intake to zero.

Dr. Nagagopal Venna's second report in February 2003. In this report Dr. Venna wrote the following. "I am seeing this patient for follow-up of intermittent pain of long-standing, across the bridge of the nose and on the forehead. On the whole, this pain has been tolerable and he has been managing well. He does find stress could bring on the pain and make it worse. He is taking Tegretol at a low dose as before and tolerating it well. He has also taken up various ways of relaxation, particularly with meditation and found them to be helpful in dealing with the intermittent moderate central upper facial pain. There are no new neurological symptoms. General health has been good. He is a professor of mathematics and also teaches Judaic studies, and travels the world. He has not found his pain to seriously interfere with his work. . . . I encouraged him to rely more on the relaxation and meditation to control the pain. . . ."

I was deeply moved by my interactions with Dr. Venna, a prince of a man whose empathy was apparent in every gesture and every word. His very presence promoted healing. This is how the sick and the broken must have felt in the presence of the Buddha and in the presence of Jesus.

I suffered from a spiritual disease. None of the doctors whom I consulted suggested that I might have been suffering from a spiritual disease. But Lama Tashi Namgyal understood:

> According to the teachings of the Buddha Shakyamuni, recorded in the *Sutra on Entering the Womb*, there are four classes of illness. . . . The third class of illness includes those for which medicines are of no use, illnesses from which one cannot recover simply through the use of medicines or other medical procedures. These illnesses, however, can be cured — and one can thereby recover one's health — through the practice of appropriate spiritual techniques taught in the buddhadharma. . . . Through such practices, the innate healing powers inherent in the basic nature of all sentient beings can be uncovered and accessed.

The truth about my pain. My headaches are a spiritual disease not curable by medication. In her article titled "Tough Teachings To Ease the Mind," the Thai meditation-teacher, Upasika Kee Nanayon, writes that one must know suffering in order to be free of it; one must let sensations, emotions, and thoughts pass without clinging or attachment; one must distinguish the concept of pain from its reality as an ever-changing energy flow not under one's control. Here is an excerpt from her teaching:

> Just don't think that *you're* what's hurting. Simply see the natural phenomena of physical and mental events as they arise and pass away. They're not you. They're not really yours. You don't have any control over them.
>
> Look at them! Exactly where do you have control over them? Whatever disease there is in your body isn't important. What's important is the disease in the mind . . . — the diseases of defilement, craving, and attachment.
>
> You can't go preventing pleasure and pain, you can't keep the mind from labeling things and forming thoughts, but you can put these things to a new use. If the mind labels a pain, saying, "I hurt," you have to examine the label carefully, contemplate it until you see that it's wrong: the pain isn't really yours. It's simply a sensation that arises and passes, that's all.
>
> . . . So when the Buddha tells us to see the world as empty, this is the way we see. The dharma is right here in our body and mind, it's simply that we don't see it — or we see it wrongly. If we

look at things with the eyesight of mindfulness and discernment, what is there to make us suffer? Why is there any need to fear pain and death? If we understand that the latching on is what makes us suffer, then all we have to do is let go and we'll see how there is release from suffering right before our very eyes.

Early warning system. My pain is an early warning system for stress. When stress is on the horizon, my nose knows.

This is how control feels. I was invited to spend a week in Dresden, Germany in October 2006 to give an eight-hour lecture series on the theory of large deviations and applications to statistical mechanics. On the Sunday before the trip — two exams to be graded, the Dresden lectures to be finished, a committee meeting and classes the next day to be prepared for, the packing to be done — how could I refuse to go with Alison to New York City to visit our daughter Melissa, son-in-law Ken, and grandson Noah? We hadn't seen them in a month, and less than a week later, I would be across the ocean, leaving Alison all alone.

On that Sunday morning, my head totally clear, I woke up at the usual time — 5:00 AM — to meditate in the usual place — the sofa in the family room, from which at 5:05 AM, just as I was starting, I heard the sound of the shower. Alison was up, way ahead of schedule, and she was going to interrupt me — though she had never done it before — telling me to get ready so that we could leave early. I moved to the guest bedroom, shut the door tight, and started again, quickly settling into the moment, trusting her. My anxiety over being interrupted had been translated into tightness in my forehead. This is how control feels. Openness in my torso as the breath breathed itself without any effort on my part. The tightness melted, and I meditated without interruption. The feeling of freedom.

We were on the road at 6:30 and reached New York City in record time. Just as I was telling Alison about my meditation adventure, the traffic approaching the Henry Hudson Bridge came to a dead stop. Inexplicably, three lanes were merging into one as the cars were being forced onto a road that would take us to God knows where. For the first time ever, I had driven to the city without my maps. Rather than directing traffic, a pair of policemen stood chatting by the side of the road, their cruiser blocking our usual route. I stopped and asked the first cop for directions, then continued on our journey, reaching Melissa's apartment an hour late. Why had the traffic been diverted from the bridge? We decided to live with the mystery and never tried to find out.

Head pain, tiredness, and energy blockage. In his book, *The Healing Power of Mind*, Tulku Thondup includes a section called "Clearing Energy Blocks" with the following chapters: "Releasing the Shackles of Tension," "Restoring the Energy of Peace and Joy," and "Nursing the Flower of Positive Energy." These words resonate with me because I'm convinced that my facial pain is caused by an energy blockage.

When the energy blockage is in my eyes or forehead, my brain often (mis)interprets it as tiredness. I can alleviate the tiredness by lying down, shutting my eyes, and trusting the wisdom of my body, which knows what to do without my intervention or control. After several minutes, by a mysterious process I cannot articulate except to say that it feels like an energy-wave rolling up my forehead, the blocked energy is released and the tiredness disappears. Is it really tiredness? Occasionally I have another experience. The blocked energy is not fully released, but jumps to a spot in my jaw, and my upper face becomes pain-free.

I had an intense experience of energy flow one evening in July 2004 when I felt extremely tired and lay down. Soon I felt something flowing through my forehead like water. It was the blocked energy that my resting had opened up and released. It flowed through my forehead, the tiredness vanished, and I was awake, once again a beneficiary of listening to my body.

When the energy blockage is in my nose, the experience is different. In that case my brain (mis)interprets it not as tiredness, but as pain, and even after I lie down, the energy blockage is never fully released. Perhaps different nerve-pathways are involved: the pressure-pathway in my eyes or forehead, the pain-pathway in my nose.

Sometimes I can feel the sensation moving between forehead and nose. Tiredness flows into pain into tiredness as the sensation navigates the landscape of my inner face, Buddhistly transcending concepts and boundaries.

None of this is an accurate description of what occurs, but I cannot find the words. Our language allows us to discuss pleasure with much more subtlety than it allows us to discuss pain. Meditation accesses a level that is beyond words and beyond conscious control. The rewards for being open to that experience are immeasurable.

In his article, "Fear, Pain, . . . and Trust," Joseph Goldstein describes bodily sensations as a fluid energy flow, which is precisely what my pain has taught me. He also validates my insight that pain can be a path to understanding the Buddha's teachings:

Meditation practice is a path of opening. To begin with, it opens us to a deeper awareness of our bodies. Usually, we have a sense of our bodies being something quite solid and fixed. But as we develop stronger mindfulness, we experience the sensations in the body as a fluid energy flow. The solidity begins to dissolve, which itself becomes a healing process.

. . . If we can open to unpleasant painful sensations, without fear, even for some moments at a time, much of the Buddha's teaching is illuminated. We gain insight into the impermanent, selfless nature of experience. When we look carefully, we see that what we call pain is a constellation of physical sensations changing moment after moment. They may all be unpleasant, but it's not a solid, unchanging thing. . . . When we feel them closely, the impression of solidity begins to break up and we see them as part of a changing flow. We also see these sensations as selfless, meaning they are outside our control.

The universality of my experience and my insights. In 1975, along with Joseph Goldstein and Jack Kornfeld, Sharon Salzberg co-founded the Insight Meditation Center in Barre, Massachusetts. Sharon and Joseph were the leaders of the first meditation retreat that I attended there during the 1980s. At that retreat Sharon told us a story that made a lasting impression on me. It concerned a journey she had taken to Asia in order to meditate with a famous teacher. When she arrived at her destination, she was ill and found meditation difficult. She expressed her disappointment to the teacher, who replied that her experience was good practice for dying. My experience with pain is good practice for dying.

Like Joseph's wisdom about pain, quoted in the preceding section, Sharon's wisdom validates my insights. It appears in her book titled *Faith: Trusting Your Own Deepest Experience*:

> When we take apart the chord of our pain, even though the experience may remain difficult, the pain becomes an alive system, with movement and variation and flux. Just as the world is breathing, the pain is breathing. It's inhaling and exhaling, and there is space between its arisings. Rather than feeling overcome and helpless in the face of a wall of pain, we can find hope, relief in that rhythm of change.

Having my insights confirmed by these two meditation teachers was a milestone in my journey of healing.

In an article written by Doctors Sun, Kuo, and Chiu, a person who suffered from severe headaches reports on the relief he found through practicing mindfulness meditation. His words could have been my own:

> While observing the change in my headache, I understood how physical sensations could be modified and controlled by mental means. When I feared a headache and tried to avoid it, I was actually bound more tightly to the pain. But when I put aside my anxious feelings, my pain and discomfort grew less. This experience helped

me to understand my body more deeply, and to sense its innate ability to adjust and recover. . . .

To meditate is to trust the innate wisdom of the body. It knows how to heal itself if we give it silence and space.

Metaphors for meditation

Meditating on the knife's edge #1. The knife with which Abraham almost sacrificed his son sits balanced inside my face. It's the same knife about which Kafka wrote "On this knife's edge we live" in his parable, "The Problem of the Laws." The knife's edge manifests itself when I meditate, a clump of sensation in the bridge of my nose. The energy of my attention emits a breath-spirit-*ruach*-wind that hovers over the knife, like the *ruach Elohim* hovering over the waters in Genesis 1:2. The knife totters. If it falls up, the sensation vanishes. If it falls down, the spirit-breath-*ruach*-wind flows into my nose channel and coagulates. I will feel it all day. If it falls up, I note it and say, "Thank you for coming and going." If it falls down, I note it and say, "Welcome, my friend. We will be spending another day together."

Meditating on the knife's edge #2. In the insight meditation that I practice, the traditional place of focus is on the breath as it flows through the nostrils. But today that is the center of the pain. As soon as I shut my eyes, it is there, not a pain, but tightness in my forehead, an energy blockage. The clouds in my mind's sky grow dark. Will the tightness cascade into my nose? Fear. If it docs, then it will stay there all day. The tightness is a leopard crouching on the knife's edge. If I remain fearful or if I follow the breath in my nostrils or if . . ., then the leopard might vault down. If I am fearless or if I follow the rise and fall of my stomach or if . . ., then it might not vault down, or then again, it might. I breathe through the paradox. As my therapist Jean Colucci taught me, the insight I gain from observing the unfolding show with equanimity far exceeds the discomfort of the pain.

Meditating on the razor's edge. Chögyam Trungpa counsels that we bring our "natural inquisitiveness" to explore that edge:

> There is a quality of fearlessness in enlightenment, not regarding the world as an enemy, not feeling that the world is going to attack us if we do not take care of ourselves. Instead, there is a tremendous delight in exploring the razor's edge.

The truths of Buddhism are actualized in the pain. The truths of Buddhism are not abstract doctrines to me, but concrete expressions of the truth that I often feel in my face. Paradoxical for many, the Buddhist teachings are made concrete by the headaches. An example is the three aspects of existence:

> *Anicca* or impermanence: the pain comes, the pain goes.
> *Anatta* or no-self: the pain has a life of its own.
> *Dukkha* or suffering: I will suffer if I try to push it away.

The truth of impermanence came home to me in a particularly graphic way on a morning in February 2005 as Alison and I were preparing to go to New York City to visit Melissa and her family. Melissa's phone call at 7:00 AM, telling us that we should be at her apartment by noon, caused a flurry of anxiety. Would we have time to stop in New Haven for coffee as we always did? Should we go straight to Melissa's apartment or first to the hotel? What if we couldn't find a parking space to unload our bags?

After we left our house, Alison was not in her usual, jovial, going-to-New-York-City mood. But I didn't say anything because I knew that the phone call was bothering her. It wasn't me. Just as we reached the highway, the energy flow in my face started to coagulate. A concept formed: headache. An accusation formed: Melissa's phone call is giving me a headache.

I have learned from the pain and said nothing. I let it go because the annoyance was minor. Why say anything that might solidify the concept of headache and cause myself to suffer? Soon the energy blockage liquefied and dissolved, the energy flowed, and my head was clear. I did all this almost instinctively, with hardly any thought.

That evening, I was reading Lama Tashi Nagyal's introduction to *Medicine Buddha Teachings* and came across the following passage concerning what the author calls "the nature of reality":

> All phenomena are ephemeral, constantly changing in the same way as the appearances within a kaleidoscope constantly change. None of these illusory appearances — including the appearances of sickness and disease, which are also mere empty appearances — has the power to cause us suffering unless we mistakenly apprehend them as real and substantial. When we misapprehend these appearances, when we take them to be real, we fixate on them and thereby cause them to solidify in our experience. This

gives them the appearance of solid, substantial reality, and then in our lives these illnesses do, in fact, become for us very real and solid, and we suffer from them.

This was precisely what I realized as Alison and I were driving to New York City. Because I handled it skillfully, what started out as a mild annoyance about our plans for the day gave me access to a deep insight. The palace of Buddhist wisdom, I realized once again, is not high on a mountaintop, but lies right under our feet, and the floor has many doors. Epiphanies do not just happen at the Grand Canyon, or when having an orgasm, or when standing before the Western Wall in Jerusalem for the first time in your life and the sun breaks through the clouds, forming a rainbow that stretches from the Judean Desert to the Mediterranean Sea and infinitely beyond. They also happen while traveling south on Interstate 91 toward New Haven early on a Saturday morning.

Mindfulness is the universal remedy. The web of Buddhist insight and wisdom is embroidered on the warp and woof of mindfulness. To be mindful is to be aware of the present moment without judgments, stories, and projections. To be mindful is to disperse the conceptual fog in which we live so that we can bring bare attention to what is happening now. To be mindful is to recognize the open, empty nature of mind. Cultivated in the practice of meditation, mindfulness illuminates our every perception, thought, and interaction. It cleanses the mind of the poisons of greed, hatred, and delusion and brings to the mind the balms of concentration, insight, and balance. In the words of Kalu Rinpoche, the great Tibetan-master, mindfulness is "the panacea, the universal remedy that in and of itself cures all delusion, all negative emotion, and all suffering."

The universal remedy? In this postmodern world ruled by relativity, incompleteness, and uncertainty, is not such a claim embarrassingly grandiose? But the Buddha is subtle and wise. His teachings do not deny relativity, incompleteness, and uncertainty but rather are based on them. As he taught, the ultimate truth about life is that there is no ultimate truth; the unshakable foundation of our existence is that there is no foundation.

These insights are reflected in the act of meditation, in which one stabilizes the mind by focusing on that which is transient: the impermanent, life-supporting, always changing and recurring breath. As the core of meditation, the breath is the atom of Buddhist teachings. The elegance of these teachings is that, in turn, they are all contained in the breath. If one attends to the breath with perfect mindfulness, then the mysteries of suffering, no-self, impermanence, illusion, and enlightenment will be revealed as direct experiences, unmediated by judgments, stories, concepts, and projections.

Rilke hints at the truth in one of his Sonnets to Orpheus:

> Breath, you invisible poem!
> A constant interchange between our clear being
> and the world space beyond our seeing
> in which I rhythmically become.
> Solitary wave whose
> gradual sea I am.

By focusing on the breath, one can change one's life, as I changed mine. Because the most radical action is to open one's heart to peace and one's mind to insight, one can also change the world by focusing on the breath, as the Buddha changed his and ours. Thus, meditation is the perfect marriage of microscopic awareness and macroscopic effect. It is a spiritual analogue of statistical mechanics, which derives the observable, macroscopic properties of physical systems from the microscopic interactions governing the molecules that constitute the systems.

Soon after I started a regular meditation practice, I wrote this poem about mindful breathing:

> The breath breathes
> Through the lattice of my concepts.
> The tightness in the forehead
> Granulates and dissolves.
> There is no I,
> Only the breath
> Balancing on the edge of itself.
> Exiting. Entering. Balancing.
>
> But I am hungry.
> My knife cuts
> The leathery flesh of the orange,
> Oozing juice onto my fingers
> That I suck clean.
> The sun explodes in my mouth.
> The sun fades.
> There is no I.

It comes to this.
When you understand the nature of the breath,
Everything will be understood.
The everything within you and without.
The nothing within you and without.
The breathing within you and without.

Permeated with impermanence. Alison and I live in a wood-frame house in a wet climate. "The nature of wood is to rot," said Victor, the carpenter I hired to do some repairs. "It's the rainwater — you can't keep it out." With his expert eye he found rot everywhere: a vertical beam under the main downspout; the rough-hewn wood of the garage; the area where the wood of the house meets the brick of the chimney; a clapboard near the front door and another clapboard holding the front lamp, split by a nail that had been driven into a knot; a fascia board over the old woodpile; the front threshold, the rot exposed when he removed the storm door in order to sand and refinish it; the bird feeder I had built for Melissa when we bought the house a quarter century ago. Victor repaired everything except for the bird feeder, which he took down. In the cracks of the rotting wood, bright green lichen was growing, sprouting tiny flowers the color of an incandescent sunset.

A piece of paper lying on a shelf near the meditation hall in the Insight Meditation Society contains the following teaching:

> All conditioned things are impermanent. Their nature is to arise and pass away. Understanding this brings the greatest kind of happiness, which is peace.

God's name Y–H–W–H is the sound of your breathing. The title of this section is taken from Rabbi Lawrence Kushner's article "Breathing." God's name Y–H–W–H is the point at which all Jewish theology begins. This name is often transliterated as Yahweh and translated as the LORD. Like Y–H–W–H, my pain "is a verb that has been artificially arrested in motion and made to function as a noun." Thus my pain is a bridge to God, its frozen energy flowing when I meditate. In *Seek My Face, Speak My Name: A Contemporary Jewish Theology*, Rabbi Arthur Green explains the dynamism and paradox of this name of God:

> By "God," of course, I mean Y–H–W–H, the One of all being.... It is to be read as an impossible construction of the verb "to be." *HaYaH* — that which was — *HoWeH* — that which is — *YiHYeH* — that which will be — are here all forced together in a grammatically impossible conflation. *Y–H–W–H is a verb that has been artificially arrested in motion and made to function as a noun.* As soon as you try to grab hold of such a noun, it runs away from you and becomes a verb again. "Thought does not grasp you at all," as the wise have always known.... Try to say anything definitional about Y–H–W–H and it dashes off and becomes a verb again. This elusiveness is underscored by the fact that all the letters that make up this name served in ancient Hebrew interchangeably as consonants and as vowels. Really they are mere vowels, mere breath. There is nothing hard or defined in their sound. The name

of that which is most eternal and unchanging in the universe is also that which is wiped away as readily as a passing breath.

To Dad, at your grave. Today, October 19, 2008, a heavy stone lifted from my heart.

In April 2000, a month before Melissa's wedding, two months after the onset of my chronic headaches, Dad made an accusation about our relationship that cut me like a knife.

After Dad died, I did not visit his grave because I could not forgive him for that accusation. After Dad died, I did not visit his grave because I could not forgive him for not repairing our broken relationship.

Dad, you died on April 8, 2001, the first day of Passover. Today, seven and a half years later, I finally visit your grave, bereft of a father but a father and grandfather myself. Today I finally forgive you for that accusation. You were sad and lonely, and your body was growing the cancer that would kill you the next year. Today I finally forgive both you and myself for not repairing our broken relationship. Thank you for giving me all that you did. Thank you for giving me the wisdom that allows me to accept that you were not able to give me everything. Dad, I love you.

And the heavy stone lifts from my heart.

Dear Ron, my brother, I express my gratitude to you for inviting me to visit Dad's grave, thus allowing me to liberate myself from the dual Egypts of my resentment and my broken relationship with our father. May his memory be for a blessing.

The pain and the rain. Early in the morning on August 1, 2004 I opened a window to hear the rain, and I turned on the ceiling fan. Then I sat down on the sofa and began to meditate. As it sometimes happens, my first perception was stabbing pain in the mid-face area. I heard the rain and the whooshing of the fan and felt the pressure in my nose and lower forehead and realized that they are all on the same level. They are all sensations, some perceived through hearing and others perceived through the mind. The sensations in my nose are my internal weather, and I have as little control over them as I have over the external weather, which today happens to be rain. The pain is not mine just as the rain is not mine. The rain and the pain, the pain and the rain both arise from impersonal causes that I cannot control. When I realized this, the pressure in my nose and forehead subsided in intensity, and I felt much better. Miraculous. No, not miraculous. When you accept the truth, the truth will set you free.

Our lack of control over the external weather is obvious. The gift of meditation is that it helps us transfer this insight about the impersonal nature of experience to our internal weather.

Experiencing the play of impersonal forces. To understand that the rain arises from impersonal causes is easy. To transfer this understanding to one's own pain requires much deeper insight. An equally challenging domain involves interactions with other people.

Although it hardly happens any more, during the spring of 2006 I had a difficult interaction with a colleague at the university. I returned to my office and jumped into my work because I did not want to deal with the emotions generated by that interaction.

Then I paused, remembering one of the deep lessons of the headache pain. Avoiding the pain, pushing the pain away, not facing the pain are aspects of dualistic thinking; accepting the pain as my own was a key step in the process of observing the impermanence of self, which in turn led to my healing. So an hour after the difficult interaction at the university, I shut my eyes and began to follow my breath.

I sat for only fifteen minutes, but those fifteen minutes changed everything. What happened was similar to what happens every time I meditate. During the first few minutes I was aware of myself breathing. It's my breath, my nose, my pain, my body. But then I breathed through the sense of self, focusing less on the breath coming through my nostrils and more on the rise and fall of the stomach, finding myself in a refuge of insight and peace, being breathed, being lived, connecting with the stillness, spaciousness, and emptiness beyond all words.

During the first few minutes of meditating in my office, I kept replaying the conversation. He said — I said — He said — I said — Why did he say that? — Why did I say that? — If only I had said something else. — Does he like me? — What if he doesn't like me?

Then all of a sudden it vanished as I breathed through the sense of self and entered a place of deeper awareness. What I saw there was momentous. I saw how impersonal the entire experience was. I saw that the conversation with my colleague was the lightning rod that allowed him to vent his own feelings, which in turn were a reaction to the impersonal forces acting on him, forces that I could not control and that had nothing at all to do with me. After fifteen minutes I opened my eyes, grateful, yet again, for the gift of meditation that transformed my difficult interaction into an experience of insight, awareness, and growth.

Street noise and meditation. Again I turn to Kafka's parable. "Leopards break into the temple and drink to the dregs what is in the sacrificial pitchers; this is repeated over and over again;

finally it can be calculated in advance, and it becomes a part of the ceremony." I live on a busy street with lots of traffic. Even when I meditate early in the morning in the back of the house, I can hear street noise. How can this be made part of the ceremony?

The cacophony of a heavy construction truck gets louder and louder, the engine roaring, the house shaking, the chaos passing, the chaos fading, peace, another truck, a motorcycle. A perfect metaphor for impermanence. One could become enlightened by this experience.

Behind the house is the music of nature: birds, a squirrel, rustling leaves, crickets, the silence in between. The silence is our Buddha nature. The street noise is the noise of our busy minds. When the street noise passes, the silence always returns. Without the noise and without the music, would we detect the silence?

Gratitude. I am grateful when I do not have a headache. That teaches me peace. I am grateful when I have a headache. That teaches me equanimity.

How I now describe myself. I now describe myself in a way I never thought I would: I am happy. I am awake.

What is my self? What is my pain? What is the purpose of my life? Why do I love mathematics? Why do I hate mathematics? Why do I resonate so strongly to the Buddha's teachings? I have given up knowing. Knowing constricts the consciousness and blocks the laser light of wisdom.

As I write this, a copy of the magazine Buddha*dharma* sits on my desk, open to the article "Mind is Buddha" by Geoffrey Shugen Arnold, Sensei:

A simple three-word koan. Or just a one-word koan: buddhanature. So deceptively simple, so easy to leave in the realm of concept, yet it penetrates to the very heart of the matter.

Not understanding it, I luxuriate in the glow of not knowing. The only ultimate truth is that there is no ultimate truth.

Two teachings that can lead to liberation. I end this chapter with teachings from two masters. In his Dharma talk on feelings Joseph Goldstein shares the following teaching:

> Whatever feelings arise, whether pleasant, unpleasant, or neutral, abide contemplating impermanence in those feelings. Contemplate the fading away, the letting go of these feelings. Contemplating thus, we do not cling to anything in this world. When we don't cling, there is no agitation. When not agitated, we personally attain nirvana.

Contemplate impermanence and the fading away and the letting go because these experiences can lead to liberation.

Kalu Rinpoche expresses his wisdom in the form of a paradox, which can liberate us by taking us beyond words:

> We live in illusion and the appearance of things. There is a reality. We are that reality. When you understand this, you see that you are nothing, and being nothing, you are everything. That is all.

8
Finding Equanimity on the Massachusetts Turnpike

> By grasping and clinging to subject and object, we prevent ourselves from recognizing the continuous display of wisdom.
> — Thinley Norbu, *White Sail: Crossing the Waves of Ocean Mind to the Serene Continent of the Triple Gems*

IT IS JANUARY 2003. I'm driving to the mindfulness-based stress-reduction program at the University of Massachusetts Medical School in Worcester, where I'm relearning how to meditate. As I approach the entrance to the turnpike in Palmer, a new experience unfolds. Traffic is backed up from the highway all the way to the toll booth as trucks and automobiles, vans and motorcycles slowly snake their way east. To put me in the mood for the class, I have been listening to a tape of Joseph Goldstein explaining the Noble Eightfold Path of Buddhism: right understanding, right intention, right speech, right action, right livelihood, right effort, right mindfulness, and right concentration.*

---

* I reconstructed Joseph Goldstein's words on this tape by quoting from his book *The Experience of Insight: A Simple & Direct Guide to Buddhist Meditation*.

> We're on this very same journey, ascending the mountain of spiritual insight. We have already discovered the secret of its invisibility: the fact that the truth, the law, the Dharma is within us, not outside of ourselves, and that we begin from where we are.

Just as Joseph is speaking these words, I enter the endless queue of traffic stretching to the horizon. My first reaction is to go on automatic pilot by turning off the tape and worrying about getting to the stress-reduction program on time. I could easily be delayed an hour or more by an unforeseen event such as an accident or construction. However, the meditation practice has taught me something. Rather than allow myself to be drawn in, I realize that Joseph's tape is the life raft to keep me from drowning in a vortex of unskillful worry and stress. I turn the volume of the tape louder and pay attention even more closely to his words:

> [R]ight understanding deals with certain natural laws which govern our everyday lives. One of the most important of these is the law of karma, the law of cause and effect. Every action brings a certain result. Things are not happening to us by chance or accident.

Joseph said "accident," the same word that the turnpike worker uses when I ask him what is causing the traffic delay. "An SUV rolled over about a mile up the road," he replies as two police cars and a screaming ambulance tear past me in the breakdown lane. I say a prayer that the driver of the vehicle is not harmed as I creep slowly forward, actually feeling calm and centered despite the ever more real possibility that I will arrive late in Worcester. I completely let go of my stress as I settle into the moment, aware that there is absolutely nothing I can do. Staying open and relaxed is by far the best way to cope.

After about fifteen minutes, I reach the scene of the accident. An SUV is being towed away. The driver, looking shaken but not badly injured, is being led to the ambulance by a policeman. All of a sudden the road opens up, the blockage of cars and trucks and vans and motorcycles miraculously disappears, and I'm on my way. This is how freedom feels, I say to myself just as Joseph explains the power and importance of generosity:

> Giving is the expression in action of non-greed in the mind. The whole spiritual path involves letting go, not grasping, not clinging, and generosity is the manifestation of that non-attachment.

I fly east on the Massachusetts Turnpike without another vehicle in sight. Both meditation practice and dealing with the delay on the turnpike are metaphors for each other: finding oneself in a blockage, letting go, finding the opening, or rather having the opening revealed in a moment of release. Dealing skillfully with the delay on the turnpike teaches me much more about stress management than I could learn in any class.

Joseph ends his explanation of right understanding with the following words, the meaning of which I continue to meditate on both in my practice and in my everyday life:

> Right understanding also involves a profound and subtle knowledge of our true nature. In the course

of meditation practice it becomes increasingly clear that everything is impermanent. All the elements of mind and body exist in a moment and pass away, arising and vanishing continuously. The breath comes in and goes out, thoughts arise and pass away, sensations come into being and vanish. All phenomena are in constant flux. There is no lasting security to be had in this flow of impermanence. And deep insight into the selfless nature of all elements begins to offer a radically different perspective on our lives and the world. The mind stops grasping and clinging when the microscopic transience of everything is realized, and when we experience the process of mind and body without the burden of self. This is the kind of right understanding that is developed in meditation through careful and penetrating observation.

I reach the stress-reduction class at 8:55 AM. On time with five minutes to spare. The homework for the day includes the following exercise:

> Make an effort to "capture" your moments during the day. Notice when you go on "automatic pilot" — when, where, etc. Can you notice times of blocking and numbing? What pulls you off center?

This is not a coincidence. There are no coincidences. Coincidence is a concept that does not comprehend the interconnectedness of every process in the universe. I take my seat, remove my shoes, shut my eyes, and begin to follow my breath.

On the road to Worcester that morning, I wake up again to the awareness that now is all I have. In his book, *Nine-Headed Dragon River: Zen Journals 1969–1982*, Peter Matthiessen articulates this insight in the context of Zen Buddhist practice:

> To practice Zen means to realize one's existence moment after moment, rather than letting life unravel in regret of the past and daydreaming of the future. To "rest in the present" is a state of magical simplicity, although attainment of this state is not as simple as it sounds. At the very least, sitting Zen practice . . . will bring about a strong sense of wellbeing, as the clutter of ideas and emotions falls away and body and mind return to natural harmony with all creation. Out of this emptiness can come a true insight into the nature of existence, which is no different from one's Buddha nature.

Why is it so difficult to see the truth? Because on the road to Worcester that morning and during every moment of our lives, the truth is in our face.

Appendix
Learning To Meditate

How is it possible to find meaning in a finite world, given my shirt and waist size?
— Woody Allen, quoted in *The Essential Crazy Wisdom* by Wes Nisker

THE MEDITATION THAT I practice is called insight meditation. It calms the mind, focuses the attention on the present moment, and leads to self-transformation. This meditation practice could help you if you suffer from physical or emotional pain; or if life is moving too fast and you find yourself always busy and your tasks fill every available moment as a gas fills a vacuum; or if you are unhappy or depressed or fearful; or if you sleep poorly; or if you are angry; or if, like Woody Allen, you are perplexed by the arduous task of finding meaning in this finite world. Or perhaps you are just curious to learn it.

Meditating is a skill, like swimming or playing the cello. Although the instructions are simple, learning to meditate takes practice and effort. However, the rewards are potentially infinite:

- Meditation calms the mind and brings equanimity.
- It teaches us to accept whatever happens with perfect trust.

- It enables us to connect with the wisdom of our bodies and the wisdom of the present moment.
- It helps us cope with pain, reduce stress, and alleviate suffering.
- It allows the innate wisdom planted within us to blossom.
- Through meditation, we heal ourselves.
- Calming our minds creates peace within us and peace for those with whom we interact.

Here are brief instructions for insight meditation. They are an expanded version of the instructions for becoming present that I give my students at the beginning of every class I teach at the university. After reading this, I ask you to spend several minutes trying to do what I suggest:

> If you would like to participate, then I invite you to sit up straight in your chair. Feel your body in the chair and your feet on the floor. Relax and be comfortable in this space. Close your eyes. Gently focus on your breath. If you are distracted by a sound, then make a mental note of that distraction. You can't change the sound or stop it, so just let it go. Similarly, if you are distracted by a thought, then make a mental note of that distraction. Let the thought float through your mind like a cloud through the sky, and let it go. When you are able to, bring your attention back to your breath. Relax into it. Keep your attention soft and precise. Let your mind become quiet by

focusing on the always changing and recurring breath. When you feel relaxed and present, open your eyes.

What happened during the time that you just meditated? If you have done it before, then you might have experienced an ease in quieting the mind and remaining in the present moment. On the other hand, if you have never meditated, then you might have been surprised to discover that the mind has a mind of its own, jumping from thought to thought, unable to stay quiet and focused. If so, then you experienced what the Buddhists call "monkey mind."

How does the quiet mind deal with distractions such as sounds and thoughts? When we meditate, we pay attention to their coming and going without getting caught in the flow. We observe, remaining nonattached. Although we normally consider sounds as being external and thoughts as being internal, as mental phenomena they are on the same level, just like pain. Eventually the distractions cease to distract, and they become part of the passing show. Wisdom and peace arise when we learn to accept them, just as we accept the rhythmic flowing of the breath. As we focus on the breath, our mental landscape expands. Personal concerns exert less pressure in the expanded space. Because the breath sustains life, focusing on it can give rise to gratitude for the miracle of being alive.

Even in the short time that you just meditated, I hope that you felt less agitated, more aware, and more present. Perhaps after meditating, you might be able to appreciate the insight that all the Buddhist teachings are contained in the breath.

If you are interested in learning to meditate, then there are several ways to begin. Numerous books on meditation practice are available, and there are many resources on the internet. The websites *http://www.dharmaseed.org* and *http://www.audiodharma.org* are particularly helpful. Some people find it easier to learn meditation from a teacher rather than from a book or an internet talk. If you live near a meditation center, then even an hour with an experienced teacher will introduce you to the fundamentals of meditation, which you can then build on in your own practice. Try to meditate regularly in a safe and quiet place at the same time each day. When you are ready, a weekend or longer retreat will help you deepen your practice, through silence, a supportive environment, and the absence of the distractions of your everyday routine. May the calm light of awareness lead to insight, transformation, and peace.

In August 2003, after three and a half years of suffering from headaches, I learned the truth about the pain at an eight-day retreat held at the Insight Meditation Society in Barre, Massachusetts. I never expected what would eventually happen of its own accord. The mindfulness cultivated by meditation blossomed from a practical technique for dealing with the headaches and the suffering into an all-encompassing approach to my life.

Since August 2003, I have continued to meditate and to exercise daily. I have also given up trying to find the meaning of life because living mindfully in the present moment without searching is so much more meaningful.

Bibliography

Abe, Masao. *Zen and Western Thought.* Honolulu: University of Hawaii Press, 1985.

Alter, Robert. *The Art of Biblical Narrative.* New York: Basic Books, 1981.

Alter, Robert. *The Five Books of Moses: A Translation with Commentary.* New York: W. W. Norton and Co., 2004.

Alter, Robert. "Kafka as Kabbalist." *Salmagundi* 98–99 (1993), pp. 86–99.

Arnold, Geoffrey Shugen, Sensei. "Mind Is Buddha." Buddha*dharma*, Spring 2005, pp. 31–33.

Banville, John. *Shroud.* New York: Alfred A. Knopf, 2003.

Bhikkhu, Thanissaro, trans. "Adittapariyaya Sutta: The Fire Sermon." Retrieved May 30, 2009 from *http://www.accesstoinsight.org/tipitaka/sn/sn35/sn35.028.than.html.*

Bhikkhu, Thanissaro, trans. "Sallatha Sutta: The Arrow." Retrieved September 15, 2009 from *http://www.accesstoinsight.org/tipitaka/sn/sn36/sn36.006.than.html.*

Blake, William. *Blake's Job: William Blake's Illustrations of the Book of Job.* Introduction and commentary by S. Foster Damon. New York: E. P. Dutton, 1969.

Cameron, Sharon. *Beautiful Work: A Meditation on Pain.* Durham, NC: Duke University Press, 2000.

Cooper, Rabbi David A. *God Is a Verb: Kabbalah and the Practice of Mystical Judaism.* New York: Riverhead Books, 1997.

Cope, Stephen. *The Wisdom of Yoga: A Seeker's Guide to Extraordinary Living.* New York: Bantam Books, 2006.

Davis, Rabbi Avrohom, trans. *The Metsudah Chumash/Rashi*, Vol. I, *Bereishis [Genesis].* Hoboken, NJ: Ktav Publishing House, 1996.

Davis, Rabbi Avrohom, trans. *The Metsudah Chumash/Rashi*, Vol. V, *Devarim [Deuteronomy].* Hoboken, NJ: Ktav Publishing House, 1996.

Dupuis, Paul and Richard S. Ellis. *A Weak Convergence Approach to the Theory of Large Deviations.* New York: John Wiley & Sons, 1997.

Easwaran, Eknath, trans. *The Dhammapada.* Tomales, CA: Nilgiri Press, 1999.

Ellis, Richard S. *Entropy, Large Deviations, and Statistical Mechanics.* New York: Springer-Verlag, 1985. Reprinted in *Classics in Mathematics* series, 2006.

Ellis, Richard S. "Full-Blown Roses." *The Lion Rampant* (Harvard University), February 1969, p. 15.

Finkelstein, Louis. "Introduction." In *Aspects of Rabbinic Theology* by Solomon Schechter. 1909 reprint edition. New York: Schocken Books, 1961.

Fox, Everett, trans. *The Five Books of Moses.* New York: Schocken Books, 1995.

Franck, Frederick. *Fingers Pointing Toward the Sacred: A Twentieth Century Pilgrimage on the Eastern and Western Way.* Junction City, OR: Beacon Point Press, 1994.

Galilei, Galileo. *The Quotations Page*. Retrieved May 30, 2009 from *http://www.quotationspage.com/quotes/Galileo_Galilei/*.

Gates, Barbara and Wes Nisker, eds. "Change the Frame, Change the Picture: A Conversation with George Lakoff." *Inquiring Mind* 21.2 (Spring 2005), pp. 6–9.

Gendler, Everett. Commentary on "Nishmat Kol Ḥay." In *Kol Haneshamah: Shabbat Veḥagim*, p. 235. Wyncote, PA: The Reconstructionist Press, 1994.

Goldstein, Joseph. "Concepts and Reality ('Big Dipper')." Dharma talk given April 12, 1988. Retrieved February 10, 2005 from *http://teach.lanecc.edu/lugenbehld/R202/handouts/Big%20Dipper.htm*.

Goldstein, Joseph. *The Experience of Insight: A Simple & Direct Guide to Buddhist Meditation*. Boston: Shambhala Publications, 1987.

Goldstein, Joseph. "Fear, Pain, . . . and Trust." *Insight Journal*, Barre Center for Buddhist Studies, Spring 2004, pp. 9–12.

Goldstein, Joseph. *Feelings: The Gateway to Liberation*, CDJG362. Wendell Depot, MA: Dharma Seed.

Goldstein, Joseph. *The Life of the Buddha*, CD3C76H. Wendell Depot, MA: Dharma Seed.

Goleman, Daniel. "The Lama in the Lab: Buddhism and Cognitive Science in Dialogue." Lecture at Smith College on December 3, 2003.

Good, Edwin M. *In Turns of Tempest: A Reading of Job with a Translation*. Stanford, CA: Stanford University Press, 1990.

Gowans, Christopher W. *Philosophy of the Buddha*. New York: Routledge, 2003.

The Great Hadassah WIZO Cookbook. Compiled by members of Edmonton Hadassah WIZO. New York: Gramercy Publishing, 1985.

Green, Arthur. *Seek My Face, Speak My Name: A Contemporary Jewish Theology.* Northvale, NJ: Jason Aronson, 1992.

Handelman, Susan A. *Slayers of Moses: The Emergence of Rabbinic Interpretation in Modern Literary Theory.* Albany: State University of New York Press, 1982.

Hanh, Thich Nhat. *Old Path, White Clouds: Walking in the Footsteps of the Buddha.* Translated by Mobi Ho. Berkeley, CA: Parallax Press, 1991.

Hanh, Thich Nhat. *Understanding Our Mind.* Berkeley, CA: Parallax Press, 2006.

Harshav, Benjamin. "Introduction: Herman Kruk's Holocaust Writings." In *The Last Days of the Jerusalem of Lithuania: Chronicles from the Vilna Ghetto and the Camps, 1939–1944* by Herman Kruk. Edited by Benjamin Harshav, translated by Barbara Harshav. New Haven: YIVO Institute for Jewish Research / Yale University Press, 2002.

"The Indra's Net: What Is It?" Retrieved November 30, 2004 from *http://www.heartspace.org/misc/IndraNet.html.*

Kafka, Franz. "The Leopards in the Temple." *Parables and Paradoxes*, p. 93. Edited by Nahum N. Glatzer. New York: Schocken Books, 1961.

Kafka, Franz. "The Problem with Our Laws." *Parables and Paradoxes*, pp. 155–159. Edited by Nahum N. Glatzer. New York: Schocken Books, 1961.

Kafka, Franz. *The Trial.* Translated by Willa and Edwin Muir. New York: Schocken Books, 1984.

Koren, Israel. "Friedrich Weinreb's Commentary on the Two Tales of Creation in Genesis." *Jewish Studies Quarterly* 6 (1999), pp. 71–112.

Kornfeld, Jack. *The Art of Forgiveness, Lovingkindness, and Peace*. New York: Bantam Books, 2002.

Krishnamurti, J. *Krishnamurti on Education*. Ojai, CA: Krishnamurti Foundation of America, 1974.

Kushner, Lawrence. "Breathing." In *The Jewish Lights Spirituality Handbook: A Guide to Understanding, Exploring & Living a Spiritual Life*, pp. 39–40. Edited by Stuart M. Matlins. Woodstock, VT: Jewish Lights Publishing, 2001.

Kushner, Lawrence. *God Was in This Place and I, i Did Not Know: Finding Self, Spirituality and Ultimate Meaning*. Woodstock, VT: Jewish Lights Publishing, 1991.

Latke. (n.d.). *Dictionary.com Unabridged (v. 1.1)*. Retrieved December 29, 2006 from Dictionary.com website: *http://dictionary.reference.com/browse/latke*.

Lew, Alan. *Be Still and Get Going: A Jewish Meditation Practice for Real Life*. New York: Little, Brown and Co., 2005.

Loy, David. *Lack and Transcendence: The Problem of Death and Life in Psychotherapy, Existentialism, and Buddhism*. Amherst, NY: Humanity Books, 2000.

Loy, David R. *Money, Sex, War, Karma: Notes for a Buddhist Revolution*. Boston: Wisdom Publications, 2008.

Mandelbrot, Benoit B. *The Fractal Geometry of Nature*. New York: W. H. Freeman, 1983.

Matthiessen, Peter. *Nine-Headed Dragon River: Zen Journals 1969–1982*. Boston: Shambhala Publications, 1985.

Michener, James A. *The Source*. New York: Random House, 1965.

Mitchell, Stephen. *A Book of Psalms*. New York: HarperCollins, 1993.

Namgyal, Lama Tashi. "Introduction." In *Medicine Buddha Teachings* by Khenchen Thrangu Rinpoche. Ithaca, NY: Snow Lion Publications, 2004.

Nanayon, Upasika Kee. "Tough Teachings To Ease the Mind." *Tricycle*, Spring 2005, pp. 34–37.

Nisker, Wes. *The Essential Crazy Wisdom*. Berkeley, CA: Ten Speed Press, 2004.

Norbu, Thinley. *White Sail: Crossing the Waves of Ocean Mind to the Serene Continent of the Triple Gems*. Boston: Shambhala Publications, 2001.

Ouaknin, Marc-Alain. *Mysteries of the Alphabet: The Origins of Writing*. Translated by Josephine Bacon. New York: Abbeville Press Publishers, 1999.

Pascal, Blaise. *Pensées*. Translated by A. J. Krailsheimer. Harmondsworth, UK: Penguin Books, 1966.

Rahula, Walpola. trans. "The Four Noble Truths." In *Radiant Mind: Essential Buddhist Teachings and Texts*, pp. 65–66. Edited by Jean Smith. New York: Riverhead Books, 1999.

Ramban (Nachmanides). *Commentary on the Torah: Genesis*. Translated by Rabbi Dr. Charles Chavel. New York: Shilo Publishing House, 2005.

Rilke, Rainer Maria. "Breath, You Invisible Poem!" In *Sonnets to Orpheus*, p. 157. Translated by Willis Barnstone. Boston: Shambhala Publications, 2004.

Rinpoche, Kalu. *Luminous Mind: The Way of the Buddha*. Translated by Maria Montenegro. Boston: Wisdom Publications, 1997.

Rinpoche, Kalu. "Quotes." Retrieved February 4, 2010 from *http://thinkexist.com/quotes/kalu_rinpoche/*.

Salzberg, Sharon. *Faith: Trusting Your Own Deepest Experience.* New York: Riverhead Books, 2002.

Scherman, Rabbi Nosson, trans. *The Complete ArtScroll Siddur.* Brooklyn: Mesorah Publications, 1986.

Scholem, Gershom. "Religious Authority and Mysticism." In *On the Kabbalah and Its Symbolism*, pp. 5–31. Translated by Ralph Mannheim. New York: Schocken Books, 1965.

Shapiro, Rami. *The Way of Solomon: Finding Joy and Contentment in the Wisdom of Ecclesiastes.* New York: HarperSanFrancisco, 2000.

Shirer, William L. *The Rise and Fall of the Third Reich: A History of Nazi Germany.* New York: Simon & Schuster, 1960.

Siegel, Ronald D. "Psychophysiological Disorders: Embracing Pain." In *Mindfulness and Psychotherapy*, pp. 173–196. Edited by Christopher K. Germer, Ronald D. Siegel, and Paul R. Fulton. New York: The Guilford Press, 2005.

Slezkine, Yuri. *The Jewish Century.* Princeton, NJ: Princeton University Press, 2004.

Smith, Jean. "Life of the Buddha." In *Radiant Mind: Essential Buddhist Teachings and Texts*, pp. 3–6. Edited by Jean Smith. New York: Riverhead Books, 1999.

Soloveitchik, Rabbi Joseph B. *Halakhic Man.* Translated by Lawrence Kaplan. Philadelphia: Jewish Publication Society of America, 5743/1983.

Spinoza, Benedict de. "On the Interpretation of Scripture." In *A Theologico-Political Treatise and A Political Treatise,* pp. 98–119. Translated by R. H. M. Elwes. New York: Dover Publications, 1951.

Steiner, George. "A Preface to the Hebrew Bible." In *No Passion Spent: Essays 1978–1995*, pp. 40–87. New Haven: Yale University Press, 1996.

Stern, Chaim, ed. *Gates of Forgiveness*. New York: CCAR Press, 1993.

Sun, Tzan-Fu, Chung-Chih Kuo, and Nien-Mu Chiu. "Mindfulness Meditation in the Control of Severe Headaches." *Chang Gung Medical Journal* 25.8 (August 2002), pp. 538–541

Sunim, Mu Soeng. *Heart Sutra: Ancient Buddhist Wisdom in the Light of Quantum Reality*. Cumberland, RI: Primary Point Press, 1991.

Tatz, Akiva and David Gottlieb. *Letters to a Buddhist Jew*. Southfield, MI: Targum Press, 2004.

Thomas, Lewis. *The Lives of a Cell: Notes of a Biology Watcher*. New York: Viking Press, 1974.

Thondup, Tulku. *The Healing Power of Mind: Simple Meditation Exercises for Health, Well-Being, and Enlightenment*. Boston: Shambhala Publications, 1998.

Trible, Phyllis. "What God Meant to Say . . ." *New York Times Book Review*, December 21, 1997, pp. 7–8.

Trungpa, Chögyam. "[OceanofDharma] Quotes of the Week: Licking Honey on a Razor Blade." E-mail from Carolyn Gimian <cgimian@suchns.com> dated May 5, 2008.

Walker, Kathryn. *A Stopover in Venice*. New York: Alfred A. Knopf, 2008.

Wallis, Claudia. "The Right (and Wrong) Way to Treat Pain." *Time Magazine*, February 28, 2005, pp. 46–57.

Waltke, Bruce K. and M. O'Connor. *An Introduction to Biblical Hebrew Syntax*. Winona Lake, IN: Eisenbrauns, 1990.

Weinreb, Friedrich. *Schöpfung im Wort: Die Struktur der Bibel in jüdischer Überlieferung*. Weiler im Allgäu, Germany: Thauros Verlag, 1994.

"When We Should Act." *Buddhas.net: An Invitation to Enlightenment*. Retrieved February 1, 2007 from http://www.buddhas.net/when.html.

Wieseltier, Leon. *Kaddish*. New York: Alfred A. Knopf, 1998.

Yellin, Tamar. *The Genizah at the House of Shepher*. Milford, CT: The Toby Press, 2005.

Zlotowitz, Rabbi Meir, trans. *Bereishis: Genesis*, Vol. 1, second edition. The ArtScroll Tanach Series. Brooklyn: Mesorah Publications, 1980.

The Zohar, Vol. III. Translated by Harry Sperling, Maurice Simon, and Paul P. Levertoff. New York: Soncino Press, 1984.

Zornberg, Avivah Gottlieb. *Genesis: The Beginning of Desire*. Philadelphia: Jewish Publication Society, 5755/1995.

Zornberg, Avivah Gottlieb. "Seduced into Eden: The Beginning of Desire." Lecture at the University of Massachusetts Amherst on May 3, 2004.

Suggested Reading

Buddhism

Easwaran, Eknath, trans. *The Dhammapada*. Tomales, CA: Nilgiri Press, 1999.

Feldman, Christina. *Silence: How To Find Inner Peace in a Busy World*. Berkeley, CA: Rodmell Press, 2003.

Goldstein, Joseph. *The Experience of Insight: A Simple & Direct Guide to Buddhist Meditation*. Boston: Shambhala Publications, 1987.

Goldstein, Joseph. *Insight Meditation: The Practice of Freedom*. Boston: Shambhala Publications, 1993.

Goleman, Daniel. *Destructive Emotions: How Can We Overcome Them?* New York: Bantam Books, 2003.

Gowans, Christopher W. *Philosophy of the Buddha*. New York: Routledge, 2003.

Hanh, Thich Nhat. *Old Path, White Clouds: Walking in the Footsteps of the Buddha*. Translated by Mobi Ho. Berkeley, CA: Parallax Press, 1991.

Johnson, Kent and Craig Paulenich. *Beneath a Single Moon: Buddhism in Contemporary American Poetry*. Boston: Shambhala Publications, 1991.

Kaza, Stephanie, ed. *Hooked! Buddhist Writings on Greed, Desire, and the Urge to Consume.* Boston: Shambhala Publications, 2005.

Kornfeld, Jack. *The Art of Forgiveness, Lovingkindness, and Peace.* New York: Bantam Books, 2002.

Loy, David R. *Money, Sex, War, Karma: Notes for a Buddhist Revolution.* Boston: Wisdom Publications, 2008.

Rinpoche, Kalu. *Luminous Mind: The Way of the Buddha.* Translated by Maria Montenegro. Boston: Wisdom Publications, 1997.

Rosenberg, Larry with David Guy. *Breath by Breath: The Liberating Practice of Insight Meditation.* Boston: Shambhala Publications, 1998.

Salzberg, Sharon. *Faith: Trusting Your Own Deepest Experience.* New York: Riverhead Books, 2002.

Smith, Huston and Philip Novak. *Buddhism: A Concise Introduction.* New York: HarperSanFrancisco, 2003.

Smith, Jean, ed. *Radiant Mind: Essential Buddhist Teachings and Texts.* New York: Riverhead Books, 1999.

Tarrant, John. *The Light Inside the Dark: Zen, Soul, and the Spiritual Life.* New York: HarperPerennial, 1998.

Tsering, Geshe Tashi. *The Four Noble Truths.* The Foundation of Buddhist Thought, Vol. I. Boston: Wisdom Publications, 2005.

Young, Shinzen. *Break Through Pain: A Step-by-Step Mindfulness Meditation Program for Transforming Chronic and Acute Pain.* Boulder, CO: Sounds True, 2004.

Jewish Spirituality

Cohen, Norman J. *Hineini in Our Lives: Learning How to Respond to Others Using 14 Biblical Texts & Personal Stories.* Woodstock, VT: Jewish Lights Publishing, 2003.

Cohen, Seymour J., trans. *The Holy Letter: A Study in Jewish Sexual Morality.* Northvale, NJ: Jason Aronson, 1993.

Cooper, Rabbi David A. *God Is a Verb: Kabbalah and the Practice of Mystical Judaism.* New York: Riverhead Books, 1997.

Davis, Avram, ed. *Meditation from the Heart of Judaism: Today's Teachers Share Their Practices, Techniques, and Faith.* Woodstock, VT: Jewish Lights Publishing, 1999.

Frankel, Estelle. *Sacred Therapy: Jewish Spiritual Teachings on Emotional Healing and Inner Wholeness.* Boston: Shambhala Publications, 2003.

Ginsburgh, Rabbi Yitzchak. *The Alef-Beit: Jewish Thought Revealed through the Hebrew Letters.* Northvale, NJ: Jason Aronson, 1995.

Green, Arthur. *EHYEH: A Kabbalah for Tomorrow.* Woodstock, VT: Jewish Lights Publishing, 2003.

Green, Arthur. *Seek My Face, Speak My Name: A Contemporary Jewish Theology.* Northvale, NJ: Jason Aronson, 1992.

Handelman, Susan A. *Slayers of Moses: The Emergence of Rabbinic Interpretation in Modern Literary Theory.* Albany: State University of New York Press, 1982.

Heschel, Abraham Joshua. *God in Search of Man: A Philosophy of Judaism.* New York: Farrar, Straus and Giroux, 1976.

Kamenetz, Roger. *The Jew in the Lotus: A Poet's Rediscovery of Jewish Identity in Buddhist India.* New York: HarperSanFrancisco, 1994.

Kushner, Lawrence. *The Book of Letters: A Mystical Alef-Bait*. New York: Harper & Row, 1975.

Lew, Alan. *Be Still and Get Going: A Jewish Meditation Practice for Real Life*. New York: Little, Brown and Co., 2005.

Munk, Rabbi Michael L. *The Wisdom in the Hebrew Alphabet: The Sacred Letters as a Guide to Jewish Deed and Thought*. Brooklyn: Mesorah Publications, 1983.

Rhine, Adam with Louise Temple. *Hebrew Illuminations*. Boulder, CO: Sounds True, 2006.

Roth, Rabbi Jeff. *Jewish Meditation Practices for Everyday Life: Awakening Your Heart, Connecting with God*. Woodstock, VT: Jewish Lights Publishing, 2009.

Shapiro, Rami. *The Way of Solomon: Finding Joy and Contentment in the Wisdom of Ecclesiastes*. New York: HarperSanFrancisco, 2000.

Slater, Jonathan P. *Mindful Jewish Living: Compassionate Practice*. New York: Aviv Press, 2004.

Wieseltier, Leon. *Kaddish*. New York: Alfred A. Knopf, 1998.

Philosophy and Science

Austin, James H., M.D. *Zen and the Brain: Toward an Understanding of Meditation and Consciousness*. Cambridge, MA: MIT Press, 1998.

Austin, James H., M.D. *Zen–Brain Reflections*. Cambridge, MA: MIT Press, 2006.

Everdell, William R. *The First Moderns: Profiles in the Origins of Twentieth-Century Thought*. Chicago: University of Chicago Press, 1998.

Lakoff, George and Mark Johnson. *Philosophy in the Flesh: The Embodied Mind and Its Challenge to Western Thought.* New York: Basic Books, 1999.

Morrison, Robert G. *Nietzsche and Buddhism: A Study in Nihilism and Ironic Affinities.* New York: Oxford University Press, 1997.

Ricard, Matthieu and Trinh Xuan Thuan. *The Quantum and the Lotus: A Journey to the Frontiers Where Science and Buddhism Meet.* Translated by Ian Monk. New York: Crown Publishers, 2001.

Rubenstein, Rheta and Randy Schwartz. "The Duplicity of Two." *Math Horizons*, April 2000, pp. 25–28.

Wigner, Eugene. "The Unreasonable Effectiveness of Mathematics in the Natural Sciences." *Communications on Pure and Applied Mathematics* 13.1 (1960), pp. 1–14.

Torah Commentary and Translations

Alter, Robert. *The Art of Biblical Narrative.* New York: Basic Books, 1981.

Alter, Robert. *The Art of Biblical Poetry.* New York: Basic Books, 1985.

Alter, Robert. *The Five Books of Moses: A Translation with Commentary.* New York: W. W. Norton and Co., 2004.

Crumb, R. *The Book of Genesis Illustrated.* New York: W. W. Norton and Co., 2009.

Ellis, Richard S. "The Book of Leviticus and the Fractal Geometry of Torah." *Conservative Judaism* 50.1 (1997), pp. 27–34.

Fox, Everett, trans. *The Five Books of Moses.* New York: Shocken Books, 1995.

Friedman, Richard Elliott. *Commentary on the Torah.* New York: HarperSanFrancisco, 2001.

Good, Edwin M. *In Turns of Tempest: A Reading of Job with a Translation.* Stanford, CA: Stanford University Press, 1990.

Halevi, Shira. *The Life Story of Adam and Havah: A New Targum of Genesis 1:26–5:5.* Northvale, NJ: Jason Aronson, 1997.

Kass, Leon R. *Beginning of Wisdom: Reading Genesis.* New York: Free Press, 2003.

Kugel, James L. *The Bible As It Was.* Cambridge, MA: Belknap Press of Harvard University Press, 1997.

Kushner, Lawrence. *God Was in This Place and I, i Did Not Know: Finding Self, Spirituality and Ultimate Meaning.* Woodstock, VT: Jewish Lights Publishing, 1991.

Steiner, George. "A Preface to the Hebrew Bible." In *No Passion Spent: Essays 1978–1995*, pp. 40–87. New Haven: Yale University Press, 1996.

Wilson, Edmund. "On First Reading Genesis." *The New Yorker*, May 15, 1954, pp. 117–144.

Zornberg, Avivah Gottlieb. *Genesis: The Beginning of Desire.* Philadelphia: Jewish Publication Society, 5755/1995.

About the Author

RICHARD S. ELLIS grew up in Boston and attended Harvard, where he majored in mathematics and German literature. He earned his Ph.D. at the Courant Institute of Mathematical Sciences at New York University. He then taught at Northwestern University and in 1975 joined the Department of Mathematics and Statistics at the University of Massachusetts Amherst, where he is now a professor. Richard has published numerous papers in mathematics and related areas and is the author of two math books (the second with Paul Dupuis), which explore the theory of large deviations in probability theory.

Richard's experiences while living in Israel in 1982 and 1986 inspired him to teach the Torah and to lead a Jewish faculty group at the University of Massachusetts Amherst. These activities led to his appointment in 1998 as an adjunct professor in the Department of Judaic and Near Eastern Studies at the University of Massachusetts Amherst, where he has taught courses on the Book of Genesis, the Book of Job, and the writings of Franz Kafka. He has also published poetry and articles on the Torah, literature, art, and anti-Semitism and the Holocaust.

Richard has lectured widely on his work in the US, Europe, and Israel. He has also had extensive experience with Buddhist meditation, having led a number of meditation groups and participated in retreats at the Insight Meditation Society in Barre, Massachusetts and the Barre Center for Buddhist Studies. His personal web page offers detailed information about his work and his interests and can be viewed at *http://www.math.umass.edu/~rsellis*.

Richard is a father, a grandfather, and a teacher, and he is married to a teacher. Besides his family, the loves of his life are many: mathematics, the Torah, Jewish and Buddhist spirituality, literature, bicycling, jazz, strong coffee, the music of Bach. Please email Richard at *rsellis.pain.truth@gmail.com* if you would like to share your experiences with pain, suffering, or healing.